HEADWAY LIFEG

D0546000

REFLEXOLOGY

Chris Stormer

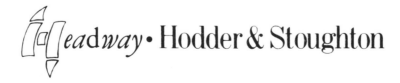

Headway • Hodder & Stoughton

I would like to express my deep gratitude to my parents, Dick and Daphne Corner, for their assistance in editing the manuscript; to Sue Risi, the photographer and Rhys Claause, the artist, for their creativity; and to Catherine Jamieson for her feet! I greatly appreciate the tremendous support and patience of family, friends, students, therapists, teachers, colleagues and my wonderful maid, Angelina, without whom I would never have found the time or the strength to complete the manuscript. I, with the publisher, would also like to thank Christina Jansen, Siobhan Chandler and Gary Ivison for the cover photograph.

British Library Cataloguing-in-Publication Data
Stormer, Christine
    Headway lifeguide: Reflexology. – (Headway
    lifeguides)
    I. Title   II. Series
    152.3

    ISBN 0–340–55594–7

First published 1992
Impression number   10 9 8 7 6
Year   1998 1997 1996

Typeset by Wearset, Boldon, Tyne and Wear

Printed in Great Britain for Hodder & Stoughton Educational, a division of Hodder Headline Plc, 338 Euston Road, London NW1 3BH by Thomson Litho Ltd, East Kilbride.

CONTENTS

For my wonderful sons

ANDREW and **DAVID**

INTRODUCTION

Cynics, and I have been one of them, would be justified in their point of view if it were not for the fact that Reflexology works time and again. Massaging the feet to improve health, and as a means of identifying the source of ill health, must seem far-fetched. However, more and more doctors have come to recognise the benefits to patients of integrating complementary health procedures, of which Reflexology is but one, into modern medical practice.

With my partner, Wendy Hunter, in a Health Centre, I conducted extensive research into Reflexology. Subsequently, as Principal of a Reflexology Academy, I learnt much of value from theses submitted by students and instructors. This knowledge, together with that gained from my earlier medical experience, contributes to the pages of this book.

Reflexology is essentially a naturally stimulating form of therapy, drawing all and sundry into its ranks of practitioners. Its mere simplicity has tempted many to exploit it, which threatens its progress and is not in the interest of the general public.

This book sets out to contribute a remedy to this situation by providing step by step guidelines in the practice of Reflexology as first conceived and practised for centuries.

Whilst there is nothing new in the concept of Reflexology – our early ancestors practised it simply by walking barefoot – methods have been adapted to contemporary needs. A significant and tangible example is the foot chart (the full colour pages 106–107 of this book), which Wendy and I developed to simplify understanding of the relationship between areas on the feet and various parts of the body.

Most people start life with the potential for good health and much illness is engendered through abuse of the body and misuse of the mind. The resulting imbalance creates a toxic build-up which inhibits the free flow of energy essential to well-being. Reflexology relaxes the body, releases an unrestricted flow of vitality and restores balance, encouraging the body's own healing system to take over. The body's recharged energy supply, ensuing from one hour of relaxation and massage of all reflexes on the feet, provides renewed physical and emotional strength to measure up to the daily demands of modern living.

Within the confines of this handbook all aspects of Reflexology cannot be addressed but it will enable everyone but the very young to take greater responsibility for his or her health.

The massage procedure is arranged according to the systems of the body. The relationship of bodily parts to the reflexes on the feet is described both in words and diagrams. A description of each organ, and how it is affected by stressful elements, is given to enhance your understanding of the dynamic effect of the Reflexology massage.

It is important to realise that each and every part of the body – physical, mental and spiritual – is interdependent within, and interacts with, the whole.

Reflexology is antagonistic to stress but, to be properly effective, massage must be applied in an appropriate manner. Consideration also needs to be given to psychosomatic symptoms so that the massage can achieve maximum effect. (See further reading, page 127: *You can heal your life* by Louise Hay.) All these aspects are covered in the step by step instruction.

This handbook is intended as a useful guide. Would-be therapists are strongly urged, in the interests of the general public, to seek qualification after a recognised course of instruction.

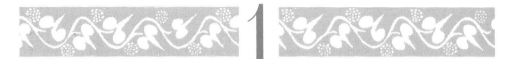

1

STRESS OR DISTRESS?

> 66 *Be grateful for the past and leave tomorrow* 99
> *in the hands of today.*

Stress is an essential element of the human constitution, although the tolerance level varies between people. Soundly based self confidence makes stress more tolerable. Indeed, by providing an element of challenge, stress is required for peak performance. The problem is not stress but our inability to cope with it.

Mismanagement of stress lies at the root of most ailments, in the form of abuse of the body. Re-establishing the lost balance of the body's energy flows is an essential therapeutic purpose of Reflexology. Its relaxing effect is as important as the physical comfort of the foot massage. Equilibrium is restored to mind, body and soul. Stress is thus no longer unwelcome. After all, there is no room for self pity. If happiness is not created now it will remain forever in the elusive future. Reflexology provides you with the strength to meet the challenge of life. This strength, combined with a desire to take charge of your own health, should encourage you to find sufficient self discipline to reconstruct the healthy lifestyle which allows you to welcome stress in the certain knowledge that you can manage it.

Regularity without rigidity and balance without obsession are the keys to health. Regular habits of eating, sleeping, working and playing, a sensible diet and avoiding extremes of thought, word or deed all contribute to a healthy body. It is then but a small step to the enjoyment of a full and useful life.

Those who persuade themselves that they are victims of stress, besieged on all sides by evil, render themselves more susceptible to disease, injury and malfunction. The risk of developing heart disease, strokes, ulcers and other serious disorders increases.

When you breathe in air, oxygen is retained and carbon dioxide released. Your food and water are digested and faeces and urine excreted. Stress, however, is progressively taken in but there is no *physical* escape valve. The resultant toxic build-up in the body's energy flows inhibits normal bodily functions. This resistance to your natural cycles of existence creates in you negativity, tiredness, tension and physical disease. Feelings of depression and unpleasant thoughts of past events lower your immunity system. Killer T cells, which fight infection, are less prolific, allowing illness and disease to gain a foothold and the cycle of self destruction has begun.

Symptoms of stress interfere with your performance and productivity, reducing the quality of your work and increasing your level of frustration. Reflexology breaks through this vicious cycle by relaxing every aspect of your body, mobilising natural healing properties from within and attending to the source of distress. A relapse can be avoided by an appropriate change of attitude and/or your lifestyle.

Symptoms of distress are more likely to occur at times of change on a personal, or wider, level; there is often a reluctance to change the familiar for the unknown. In such circumstances strife can develop within the family which family members extend to the world at large. And the unbridled materialism of many societies often pressurises people to compete for false goals in the mistaken belief that 'rich means happy'. In the process, personal integrity is eroded and a sense of proportion is lost. 'Burnout' and disillusionment are likely to follow. For Reflexology to have a lasting effect you need the will to seek 'things of value'.

Stress may, of course, be induced by events over which you may never have direct control. In this category are the fears and worries about current events happening half a world away or about the general future. This stress is a real but 'self-inflicted wound' which foot massage alone cannot heal. You need to find the strength to adopt a positive attitude.

No matter the cause, stress resists the flow of life forces within the body and drains it of its inner resources. The resultant internal pressure deprives bodily organs and cells of essential life forces. Relaxation, brought on by Reflexology, revitalises sluggish blood flow and re-establishes a state of balance.

In other words, by relieving the body of physical burdens, Reflexology opens the way and provides the strength to move on to pastures new. The benefits derived from regaining and retaining control of your mind and emotions are inestimable.

There is now greater awareness of the super-conscious, otherwise known as the spirit, which is pure and at peace with creation. It represents 'goodliness' (godliness) and is personalised as the God within. The subconscious is the soul which stores beliefs and principles engendered and conditioned throughout life. Experiences, impressions, fear, anger and guilt are buried at this level to colour, distort and segregate the conscious mind's perception of the super-conscious. The soul represents the whole spirit (the 'holy spirit').

Imagine the sun as the super-conscious and sunglasses to be the subconscious; the mind's eye will perceive the sunlight to be less bright than it really is and so the body will respond accordingly. Such filtration distorts and gives rise to mental conflict, through 'mind talk', making clear decision difficult. The battle within is between the soul and the spirit. The practice of Reflexology entails the need to be aware of the distinction between the ego of soul and the purity of spirit.

The conditioning of your mind and body throughout life by parents, teachers, clergy, peers and so on all contribute to your personality. In the normal way, everyone has the gift of choice: difficult though it may be, it is essential to let go of the ego and its lifelong belief patterns in order to release internal turmoil and avoid conflicts of thought, word and deed.

Reflexology is a positive step in releasing the mind from its shackles. You become yourself and find that there is room for love to the exclusion of ill health. Love, the creative force of life, banishes the conflict brought on by fear, anxiety, anger, greed, selfishness, discontent and other root causes of distress.

> Sorrow is the lack of joy;
> Darkness, lack of light;
> Illusion, lack of truth;
> Ignorance, lack of knowledge
> Fear, lack of love and security.

'Fear knocked at the door, faith opened it and no one was there.'
An old Chinese proverb

2

THE ROLE OF REFLEXOLOGY

> **66** *The body is one of our most precious* **99**
> *possessions.*

The human form

Your body demands little care other than love, nourishment, warmth and protection, yet many have ceased to recognise the vibrations of its natural requirements. Negligence can cause it to become inefficient and break down, but it automatically tries to fix itself, seeking attention only when it requires assistance. At this stage many entrust their bodies and lives to others. In so doing they rely on other people to provide for their health, happiness, well-being and security instead of seeking the answer within themselves.

A lively, balanced and constant interaction between all the cells within a relaxed body is a prerequisite for health. By its nature your body continually strives to be healthy and sickness is a manifestation of its attempt to ward off deterioration and dis-ease. Instead of fighting and suppressing disease, it is important to work with the dis-ease by understanding why it has occurred.

Dis-ease and discomfort are ultimately the result of persistent strain and tension causing deprivation of vital forces. Just as a plant will wilt, malform, discolour or become prone to disease through lack of sunlight, water or nutrients, so it is with the body. Malformed and diseased cells appear, as in the case of cancer.

Physical tension, triggered off by emotional 'stress', affects specialised tissues differently.

Nervous tissue

This tissue becomes very irritable, agitated, ultra sensitive and highly strung, causing it to over-react to relatively mild stimuli. Irritation in one part of the body has a widespread effect due to the overall distribution of nerve cells and fibres.

Muscular tissue

Muscular tissue is alerted and tenses as it prepares to resist threatening situations. It refuses to relax and at the least provocation will go into spasm. Great strain is placed on the already taut ligaments and tendons, making them prone to injury. Blood vessels are squeezed, in some cases, to obliteration. Their reduced capacity limits the amount and the speed of the blood flow, depriving the cells of vital components and allowing the build up of toxic wastes.

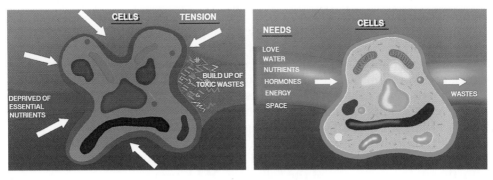

Deprived cell   *Healthy cell*

Mucosa

Mucosa increases its secretion in an attempt to flush out irritating foreign bodies that aggravate its highly sensitive lining. Its angry reaction causes swelling and redness.

The composition of an organ will determine the type of symptoms it displays when distressed. The stomach, for example, has all three of the above types of tissue and becomes both irritable and tense, with an increased outpouring of gastric secretion. For this reason merely going straight to the site of discomfort will only give temporary relief since the symptom and not the cause has been dealt with.

Reflexology recognises the marvellous recuperative ability of the body and encourages its repair work as it continually replaces used up and worn cells with fresh new material from the blood. The body constantly changes 98 percent of its atoms every year and its DNA, at the level of the atoms, every couple of months. (See Further Reading, page 127.) Red blood cells are replaced every 120 days, the skeleton every few months, the liver cells over several weeks, the stomach lining every few days, and skin cells every month, which means that even the most diseased and damaged organ has an opportunity to reproduce itself favourably *provided* there are healthy environmental conditions.

Reflexology speeds up the removal of waste materials which would otherwise poison the body and provide a breeding ground for diseased conditions. Germs do not thrive in clean, healthy conditions.

The benefits of Reflexology

Virtually everyone enjoys and benefits from Reflexology. Once internal communication and attunement have been re-established within the body, it becomes instinctively more difficult to abuse the body.

Relaxation is a prerequisite for health. Reflexology massage is capable of inducing the alpha state of relaxation, which unclutters the mind and opens it to tranquillity. The alpha state is the level of consciousness between wakefulness and sleep. It is the most serene level at which healing can effectively take place.

Initial response to the Reflexology massage varies, although ultimately there should be a life-giving surge of vitality and well-being with the overall effect extending to the mind and subconscious. People expect a quick recovery, but it is not sensible to believe that a one-off massage will correct problems that have been present and developing over many years. Your response is not related to the severity of any disorders but to your faith in your body's own healing abilities. All reactions are considered positive since they indicate that the body is actively trying to expel unwanted toxins and so-called 'side effects' are generally shortlived. One or more of the following **MAY** occur:

- skin eruptions
- minor skin rashes
- increased perspiration
- loss of body heat
- mild cold
- profuse nasal discharge
- increased secretions from the pharynx and bronchi
- post-nasal drip
- sore throat
- coughing
- increased phlegm
- sneezing
- watery eyes
- nausea
- vomiting (especially if you are on medication)
- flatulence
- increased bulk, volume and frequency of stools
- diarrhoea
- acidic, irritable vaginal discharge
- increased urine
- change in the odour and colour of urine
- extreme thirst (indicating the need to flush the system through with purified water)
- awareness of feelings
- alteration in sleep patterns eventually leading to deep, refreshing sleep
- more noticeable dreams
- increased awareness of feet and later bodily needs.

Reflexology massage relieves congestion, aids circulation, relaxes muscles, calms overactivity in any part of the body and stimulates underactivity. It improves cooperation and coordination between the bodily systems.

3

MASSAGE TECHNIQUE

66 *The lighter the touch, the greater the benefit.* **99**

The massage

Reflexology massage can be as refreshing and exhilarating for the giver as it is for the receiver! Contrary to belief it does not require a great deal of physical strength. As the 'giver' of the massage you will simply be activating healing forces within the recipient's body. To view your role otherwise assumes for you too great a responsibility. **The massage you give should *not* be painful**. To distress a 'stressed' body further inhibits the free flow of energy.

The role of the hands and feet

Interaction between the hands of the giver and feet of the receiver opens up a two way communication. Initially the hands actively give and the feet passively receive, but these roles are constantly reversed as the feet give back messages about the owner's internal environment whilst the hands receive them and respond accordingly. This process provides a vital feedback.

Society has suppressed much natural expression through touch because of sexual connotations. Yet touch is essential for optimum health, early physical and emotional development, emotional release, and for a feeling of security and love.

The giver's attitude

Accept recipients for what they are; offer no criticism, judgement or advice. If they need to talk before or after the massage give them the opportunity to do so. Assist them by asking pertinent questions such as: 'How do *you* feel about that?' and 'What do *you* believe is the solution?' because they invariably know the answers but may not be consciously aware of this. Their thoughts and feelings are put into context through expression, and the burden eased.

Important aspects

- The right side of the body is reflected onto the right foot and the left side onto the left foot.
- Always work from the receptive and receiving left foot to the giving and outgoing right foot.
- The sequence involves massaging both halves or pairs of organs and glands for a more balancing effect. As the body relaxes it lengthens, so if one side is more relaxed than the other there is a temporary but unpleasant feeling of lop-sidedness.
- The creative right side is positively fiery and represents masculinity, whilst the logical, analytical left side is negative, cooler, and represents feminity. Conflict with another person or with a particular aspect of one's personality is immediately reflected by tension in the relevant foot. A man at loggerheads with a woman will have a rigid left foot! Many a divorced woman in the unenviable position of being house-keeper, mother and father to the children, taxi driver and breadwinner, experiences tremendous inner turmoil between the masculine and feminine aspects of her personality as reflected by the feet.
- Every bodily cell and atom has positive (male) and negative (female) qualities.
- Where possible use the right hand on the left foot and vice versa. Many organs overlap in the body and likewise in the feet.
- The toes, for example, contain eye, ear, nose, mouth, sinus, teeth, gum, and throat reflexes in a relatively small area, so they have been spread out through the little toes!
- All major organs, blood and lymphatic vessels are in the centre of the body and so the massage should always progress from the outer (lesser) aspect of the feet towards the inner (greater) aspect and from the tip of the feet towards the body so that toxins can be flushed away by the lymphatics.
- When working one reflex it is possible to gain secondary access to another. For example, whilst massaging the back reflex on the top of the foot, you are also gaining access to the lungs, heart and breasts.
- Concentrate on taut, bubble-like swellings, 'gritty' deposits, or 'flabby' areas as you feel them. They are the congested, tense or sluggish areas.
- Extra bones or glands, crushed vertebrae, transplants, removal of bones, scar tissue or any other physical deviation are all reflected in the feet. Stiffness in the body is rigidity in the feet. If the feet can be loosened tension in the body is released.
- The colour and skin temperature of the foot indicate the circulation of the body.
- If a toe or part of the foot has been amputated, massage as though it is still present because the energy flow should still be intact, or can be released if trauma was experienced.
- The massage should be given one hour before medication, when the body is most vulnerable.
- **Plenty of *purified* water must be taken for at least 24 hours after the massage** to assist the body in flushing out its toxins.

Practising basic technique

The gentle massage is based on the homoeopathic principle of the weaker the dosage, the more potent the effects. In Reflexology the lighter the touch, the greater the benefit. Too much pressure undermines the incredible healing ability that everyone possesses.

Experience the energy flow by holding your hands, palms facing, fractionally apart, and feel a vibrating heat with a tingling sensation. (If it is not immediately evident, don't be concerned; it will come.) Move the hands backwards and forwards, as though playing an accordion. There will be a magnetic pull and your palms will feel as if connected by billions of invisible strings. This healing potential becomes more potent with increasing awareness.

Keep your touch light at all times, even if the receiver implores you to increase the pressure. People become addicted to harmful elements, such as nicotine, alcohol and caffeine and the need to feel pain can be the manifestation of a belief in self punishment. A person feeling deprived of love may initially be uncomfortable with the sincerity of the massage but will eventually thrive on the gentle approach.

Practise the following techniques on the hand first. Vary the pressure so that the differing potencies and effects can be experienced.

The compression massage or caterpillar walk

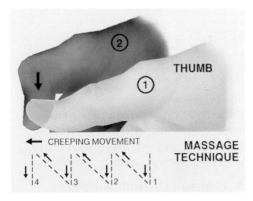

1 Place the pad of the thumb against the skin's surface towards the edge of the palm so it is pointing towards the centre.

2 Rock the thumb gently forwards onto its fleshy tip. This is the active and most stimulating phase of the movement.

3 Roll the thumb back onto the pad. This is the passive or resting phase. Repeat step 2 and continue alternating the active and passive sequence so that the thumb moves rhythmically **forward** all the time.

Footnotes
● Life is a progression and the thumb should always move forward.
● The pressure and pace should vary throughout the massage. A very tense area requires an extremely light, soothing movement. A flabby, slack area needs a firmer, more invigorating movement. Some areas may need both! You will instinctively learn to interpret the recipient's needs.
● It is easier to feel congestion and blockages by skimming the surface.
● The caterpillar movement reawakens the body and flushes energy through it. If the energy meets resistance it is immediately

reflected back to the foot. The force of the rebounding energy against the skin determines the degree of sensitivity felt in the foot and will be unnecessarily painful if the pressure is too great.

The lymphatic drainage or 'milking'

1 Keep the pad of the thumb resting gently against the skin's surface on the palm.

2 Apply gentle pressure whilst moving the thumb forward as though squeezing a tube of toothpaste! It can either be a long continuous movement or a progressive movement of smaller strokes.

Footnote
● The milking movement always follows the caterpillar walk to flush toxins through the lymphatic reflexes.

The 'healing' or 'feathering' movement

1 Use both thumbs or two fingers. This time you will need to practise on your foot.

2 Very lightly brush the surface of the skin with one finger (or thumb) followed by the other, in small stroking movements, over and over again, until you acquire a flowing affect.

3 Always move in tiny strips towards the body.

Footnotes
● This is extremely soothing and healing particularly on the nerves.
● It should always be at the end of each sequence.
● Use liberally on the nervous and endocrine systems, as well as on tense, congested areas.

Creating the right atmosphere

Although Reflexology can be done anywhere at any time, a peaceful, subdued atmosphere is best with light music playing softly in the background. Mozart's music has a healing effect on the mind and body. For the best results you should start your massage treatment as follows:

1 Soak the feet in water with a drop of peppermint and/or lavender essence, or with a sprig of fresh peppermint and lavender, to relax and cleanse the feet. It will cool hot feet in summer and warm cold feet in winter. A foot spa helps.

2 Familiarise the recipient with the workings of Reflexology if they are without previous experience and warn them of possible after effects.

3 If any of the following are experienced, reassure the recipient that their body is responding beneficially.

● A warm glow as the energy re-establishes its path.
● An inclination to sleep which should be encouraged.
● A state of euphoria.
● A floating and spreading sensation as tension is released and the body expands.

● A possible heaviness as the body relaxes.

● A shooting sensation as blockages are released.

● A dull, aching sensation as the blockage is being massaged.

● Temperature extremes as the energies reorganise themselves.

● Twitching, jerking and tingling throughout the body as the energies re-establish their paths.

● An immediate reaction in the body such as flushing of the skin, mild abdominal cramps, a postnasal drip (as the mucus trickles down the back of the throat), coughing, or a full bladder.

4 There should be **no** conversation during the massage. Talking conjures up images in the mind causing physical reactions within the body. Disturbing thoughts unconsciously tense muscles, and the heart rate increases.

5 To allow the energies to flow freely both giver and recipient should remove shoes, jewellery and tight clothing.

6 Position the recipient comfortably on a reclining chair with the feet on a pillow or on a bed with one pillow under the head and at least two under the knees. Increasing the number of pillows **under the knees** helps in the case of a back problem. Cover the body with a light sheet in summer and warm blankets in winter to retain the heat as body temperature automatically lowers with relaxation. It may be necessary to add a blanket during the massage.

7 The recipient should lie straight, with arms outstretched at the sides, preferably with the palms facing upwards to allow for the free flow of energy. If the fists are clenched, provide smooth pebbles or two pieces of rose quartz to hold. These should be held gently against the solar plexus at the end of the massage.

8 As the giver, seat yourself comfortably with the recipient's feet at chest level, keeping your legs and knees slightly apart, your back straight with your shoulders, neck and jawline relaxed. It is essential to remain relaxed so that your energies flow freely and unrestricted and to prevent the draining of your own energies.

9 Uncover the feet and gently embrace them in both hands.

10 Both giver and receiver should close their eyes and take in nine deep breaths, holding onto the inhaled air for a few moments and squeezing out every particle of air on expiration. Allow your bodies to relax and let go. Only the giver should then open the eyes. If either of you are having difficulty in relaxing, yawn to relax the facial muscles and release the jawline.

11 Avoid using oils and creams, which create a barrier and make the thumb slip. If really necessary use a light powder particularly on feet and hands that perspire easily.

12 You are now ready to begin the warm up. The whole massage should last approximately an hour.

The warm up

1 Leave the right hand on the left foot, and bring the left hand to join it. Using both hands gently stroke the top of the left foot towards you for a few seconds. (This is the only time that the massage is in this direction.) Place the left hand on the right foot, bring the right hand over to join it, and repeat the **stroking** movement.

a few seconds. Place the left third finger on the edge of the outer right ankle, and then the right third finger on the edge of the inner right ankle, and repeat the **circular** movement.

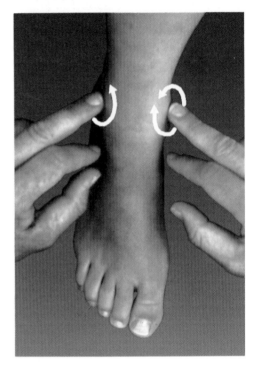

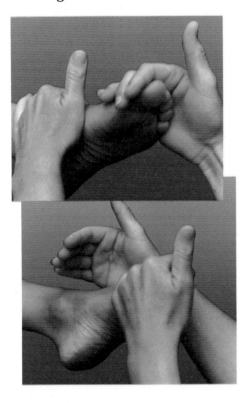

2 Place the right third finger on the edge of the outer left ankle and then the left third finger on the edge of the inner ankle of the same foot. Hardly touching the skin's surface, slowly make circular movements around both ankles for

3 Rest the mound at the base of the right thumb against the hollow below the left outer ankle, and then the mound at the base of the left thumb against the hollow beneath the left inner ankle. Without moving position, move the hands backwards and forwards to shake and loosen the ankle. The more relaxed you are the greater the movement! Repeat on the right foot with the base of the left thumb against the outer hollow and that of the right against the inner hollow. Repeat the **ankle shake**.

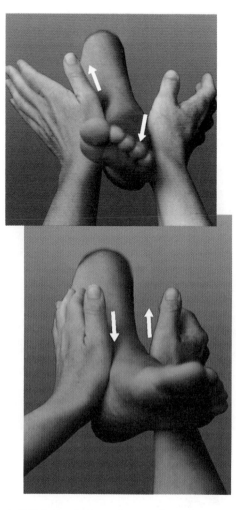

5 Place one hand under the left ankle with the other resting on top of the foot. Making sure that the recipient is totally straight, gently pull with one smooth, continuous movement using the lower hand until the spine can be seen to straighten and open up. With the upper hand in alignment with the foot, stretch the foot down as far as it will go. Repeat the **spinal stretch** on the right foot.

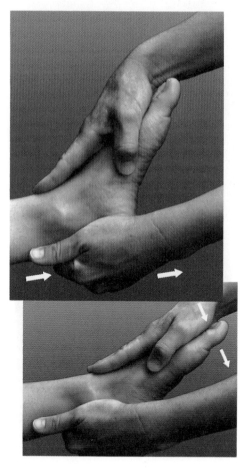

4 With both hands gently massage up and down the sides of the left foot and then repeat the **foot rub** on the right foot.

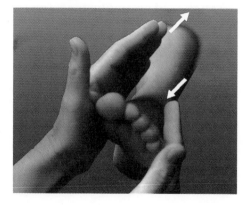

6 Hold the left toes back with the left hand, and use the flat surface between the knuckles on the right hand to massage the sole of the left foot, from the base of the toes to the tip of the ankle, working from the outside to the inside of the foot. Repeat the **knuckle rub** on the right foot with the left hand, whilst the right hand holds back the toes.

7 Using the heel of the left palm gently rub under the curve of the left instep, applying slightly more pressure on the downward rub towards the body and just brushing the skin's surface as you rub towards yourself. Repeat the **spinal rub** with the heel of the right hand on the right instep.

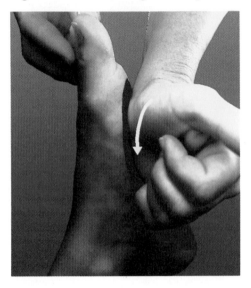

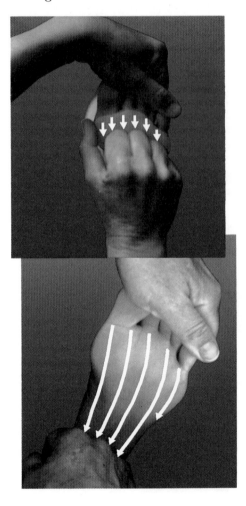

8 You are now ready to proceed to the central nervous system. (See page 25.)

Footnote
● The nervous and endocrine systems between them co-ordinate and control all bodily processes and so should always be massaged immediately after the warm-up.

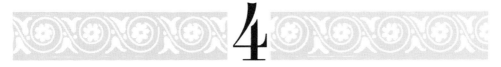

4

THE NERVOUS SYSTEM

Essential for survival, the nervous system provides a prodigious
communications network by which every part of the body – physical,
mental and emotional – is co-ordinated and controlled. It calmly
manages the intricate task of receiving and reacting to the flood of stimuli
that continually bombard the body.

Position in the body
Nerves and nerve cells infiltrate
every part of the body.

Position on the feet
Reflexes are present throughout
the feet.

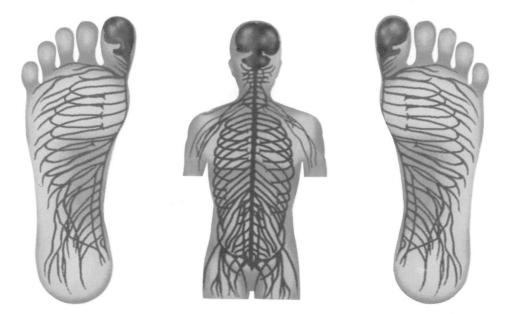

Characteristics

The *Central Nervous System* is the main processing unit of the body from
which the *peripheral nerves* radiate. 'Incoming' *sensory nerves* are
concentrated on the skin's surface, and in the organs of touch, smell,
hearing and sight to register advantageous and disadvantageous stimuli
from the internal and external environment. They release sensual
impulses to the brain for processing so that appropriate responses can be
made. A steady flow of these unperceived impulses is essential for the
maintenance of your body's vital processes.

The 'outgoing' *motor nerves* relay commands from the brain to the muscles, or cells, to make specific movements, either consciously or automatically. Automatic motions subconsciously maintain stability within and control respiration, circulation, digestion, excretion, and sexual cycles.

Effects of 'stress'

Impending danger alerts your involuntary (autonomic) nervous system to constrict blood vessels, raise blood pressure and accelerate heart beat in readiness for a greater expenditure of energy. Although beneficial in the short term, this exhausts the body and has detrimental effects if prolonged. The vice-like grip of tension deprives nerves of essential life forces with a resultant build-up of toxins. This irritates the nerves and hampers their effectiveness, which can lead to nervous disorders.

Reflexology acts as a stabiliser, and strives to protect and conserve bodily resources.

Reflexology procedure

Peripheral nerves are widespread throughout the whole body and receive continual stimulation when both feet are fully massaged properly. However, it is first necessary to pacify the whole body through the central nervous system, which requires individual attention and is massaged first.

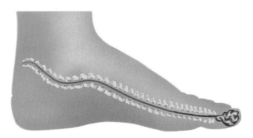

The central nervous system

The central nervous system initiates and regulates all physical and mental bodily processes, essential for survival. The brain is the mastermind and personifies the inner self and acts as its consciousness.

Characteristics

Both mind and body are nourished by thought, word and deed to greatest benefit when they exist in a perfect state of equilibrium. A reciprocal relationship exists between the body, which relies on the nervous system for survival through mental and physical activity and on the brain, which depends upon the body for a rich supply of essential life forces and for the removal of toxic or foreign substances. All are controlled from the centre of the nervous system, the brain.

A healthy brain differs from the rest of the body in that it is only capable of minimal rhythmic expansion and contraction. Its solidarity and relative immobility are ensured by the protective helmet of 20 cranial bones and disturbances of any kind is manifest in a headache or migraine.

Its wrinkled structure allows an enormous amount of brain surface to be crammed into a relatively small area. The grey matter, on the surface of the brain, accommodates the more sophisticated centres and is richly endowed with nerve cells. Immediately below is the thicker white matter with millions upon millions of nerve fibres which connect various parts of the brain and transmit almost 1000 messages per second.

The brain's healthy appetite demands about one fifth of the body's nutritional requirements, depending on the person's activities. Even a brief interruption in the supply will cause fainting. Unconsciousness occurs after ten seconds of deprivation and damage or death after a few minutes, because there is no room for storage of essential nutrients. Narrowing or calcified brain arteries lead to a gradual loss of intellect and reasoning.

Life force within the human brain has feelings, expressed through creative and/or destructive thoughts, which contribute to the wealth of images. These images are constantly conditioned by fresh thoughts which determine the nature and intensity of emotion.

The conscience and the power of reasoning mould actions and reactions to the environment and combine to develop the unique characteristics of each person. Life's experiences cannot be the same for every person or group of people, which emphasises the need to treat everyone as an individual.

The *cerebrum* initiates emotional response and its continual activity, even during sleep, demands up to 20 percent of the oxygen supply. As the seat of intelligence and memory it is responsible for perception, thought and decisions. The right side of the brain is artistic and creative, whilst the left is the logical and analytical. People have a tendency to use one side more than the other creating an unnatural imbalance.

The *hypothalamus* at the base of the brain is vital for co-ordination and control of all essential life processes, and immediately detects emotional changes.

The *brainstem* is the root of the brain and contains the *midbrain* which is continually alert to danger. It links the sensations of touch, pressure, temperature and pain to the more sophisticated centres. Some reflex muscle activity, such as blinking, is governed by the midbrain.

The *cerebellum*, or 'little brain', bulges behind the brainstem and has trebled in size over the last million years. Its main concern is to adjust orders from the cerebrum regarding posture, muscle tone and the co-ordination of muscular movement.

The *spinal cord* extends from the base of the brain to the lower back. Over 900,000 of the million nerve fibres cross over at this point so that each side of the brain controls the opposite side of the body. Throughout its length it gives off nerves in pairs to the rest of the body until it tapers off in the coccyx.

The spinal cord serves mainly as a reflex centre, and transmits impulses. A spinal reflex is an automatic, unlearned response which allows you to avoid potentially harmful situations.

The *solar plexus*, situated beneath the diaphragm, is a source of vital force and physical energy, with solar or sunlike properties. As a centre of feelings and emotions it is very important in Reflexology. Nerves radiate from its vibrant core forming a network of sympathetic ganglia supplying the abdominal organs; hence it is known as the 'abdominal brain'.

Effects of 'stress'

Creative thoughts and ideas are invariably crowded out by fear and anxiety. A dull mind inhabits a sluggish body, which is more susceptible to illness and disease, whilst a lively, inquisitive mind fills the body with vitality and enthusiasm.

From the time of conception and during the first few years of life, the brain stores a multitude of impressions for referral throughout life. Constant criticism and unreasonable restriction engenders resentment and lack of confidence. The resultant distortion later affects reasoning, thought patterns and relationships as well as physical and emotional well-being. It is exacerbated by parental, peer and social pressures. Such outdated or distorted information can be modified, changed or thrown out, releasing the brain so that it can begin to realise its incredible' potential. Parents *can* thus avoid the mistakes of their forebears in the upbringing of their children.

Belief systems are given value by their initiator, and when these are threatened anger is unleashed. Tension arising from resentment, frustration, anger and such, as a result of suppression and imposed conformity, causes the back muscles to contract and, over a period of time, the spine to curve. If the muscles on one side are more tense than on the other, the spine develops a sidewards kink and nerves are likely to be pinched. Postural balance is upset. Increased pressure on abdominal organs due to forward curvature causes undue compression, whilst backwards curvature, lordosis, strains the abdomen beyond natural limits.

Psychosomatic aspects

Boredom, anger and frustration give rise to the acute and chronic ailments of the body, often imposing physical restrictions. Headaches arise from a deep fear or anxiety. Constant headache sufferers tend to be very hard on themselves and many lack self confidence. Migraine headache sufferers harbour built-up resentment at being pushed around by others, or they may consistently resist the flow of life forces.

The spine represents flexibility and the support system of the body, and is closely related to back problems. Neck stiffness indicates a rigidity of ideas, or a means of denying knowledge of what is going on behind one's back. The upper back supports emotions and problems can arise when there is no emotional support or if a person is feeling burdened with responsibility. Guilt is tucked into the small of the back, whilst finances support the base of the spine. Continual thoughts of money tend to cause lower back pain. An inability to trust the flow of life's processes can result in curvature of the spine.

Reflexology procedure

For the purpose of massage the central nervous system is divided into sections, each of which is massaged individually on each foot, always working from the left foot to the right foot.

The brain

Position in the body
Upper part of the head.

Position on the feet
The reflex occupies the upper half of the pads on the big toe, however, at this stage, the whole pad is massaged to incorporate the face and sensory reflexes.

Reflexology procedure

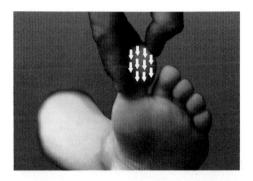

1 Support the left big toe with the left hand, leaving the pad exposed.

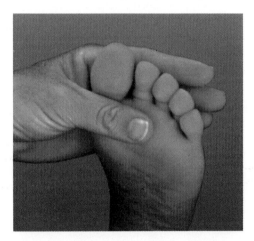

2 Place the right thumb on the right tip of the left big toe with the thumb facing downwards.

3 Caterpillar walk (see page 15) from the tip, down the inside edge of the big toe to the crease across the base of the pad.

4 Caterpillar this strip, from top to bottom, another 3 to 4 times.

5 Continue to massage in vertical strips, caterpillaring each strip at least 3 to 4 times, and progress across the pad of the big toe, until you reach the other side.

6 Place the right thumb back on the right tip of the big toe and milk the vertical strips, 2 to 3 times each (see page 16).

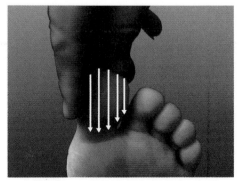

7 Use both thumbs or two fingers to heal, (or lightly caress) the whole area downwards, moving from lesser to greater (see page 16).

8 Keep the right hand on the left

foot as you place the left hand on the right foot. Once contact has been established, take the right hand over to the right foot. *It is essential to maintain contact* with one hand at all times throughout massage to maintain the energy flow.

9 Supporting the right toe with the right hand, place the left thumb on the left tip of the right toe, with the thumb facing downwards, and caterpillar vertically down the inside edge of the toe, 3 to 4 times.

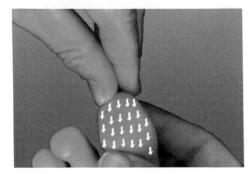

10 Repeat steps 5 to 9 on the right toe using the left thumb instead of the right.

Footnotes
● Concentrate on the brain/head reflexes when congestion or small gritty deposits are felt and for the following: headaches, nervous disorders, sinusitis, eye, ear or nose problems, acne, jaw tension, mouth related disorders, hormonal imbalances, poor temperature control, unsatisfactory eating patterns, imbalanced metabolism, poor muscle tone or reflex action, poor co-ordination, dizziness, loss of balance, hypertension or hypotension, sexual abnormalities, pain control and postural disorders.
● Massage this area for longer to treat depression, emotional distress; poor self image; stubbornness; and on those who are clinging to outdated belief structures.

The midbrain

Position in the body
Back of the head at the base of the skull.

Position on the feet
The reflexes are on the edge of the big toes, between the extreme tips of the big toes and the bony prominence midway down the side.

Reflexology procedure

1 Support the left big toe with the right hand as shown below.

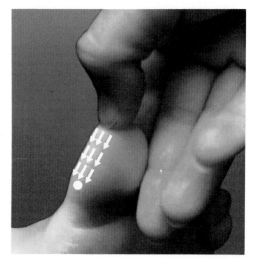

2 Use the right thumb to caterpillar in the 3 strips from the tip of the big toe to the lower part of the bony prominence midway down the outer edge of the left big toe. Repeat 3 times to complete 9 strips.

3 Still supporting the left big toe, use the right thumb to milk the 3 strips from the tip of the toe to below the bony prominence. Repeat this movement several times, depending on the amount of congestion.

4 Remove the supporting hand and use the thumbs or fingers of both hands to feather stroke the strips from the tip to the bony prominence.

5 Maintain contact as you transfer your hands over to the right foot.

6 Repeat the above procedure using the left thumb, whilst the left hand supports the right foot.

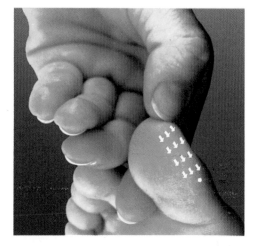

7 When you have finished move the hands over to the left foot keeping a point of contact at all times.

Footnote
• Concentrate on the midbrain reflex if there is any congestion or gritty deposits or for endocrine, circulatory, respiratory or muscular imbalances.

The cervical vertebrae

Position in the body
The neck region from halfway down the back of the head (where there is a bony knob) to the prominent bone at the base of the neck.

Position on the feet
The reflex extends from the bony prominence midway down the inner aspect of the big toes to the bony prominence at the base of the big toes.

Reflexology procedure

1 Support the left big toe with the right hand. Repeat the procedure as for the midbrain but caterpillar over **both** prominences.

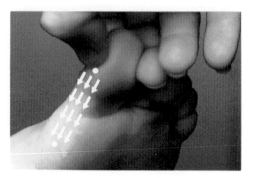

2 Having completed the left cervical reflex move the hands over to the right foot, maintaining contact.

3 After massaging the right foot place the hands, one by one, on the left foot.

Footnote
● Concentrate on the cervical reflex for rigidity of the neck or thought process. Tension tends to build up in this area, manifesting itself as congestion. If the neck is injured gritty deposits, which appear to crumble, are felt. Apply very light pressure.

The spinal cord

Position in the body
The spinal cord runs through the vertebral column from the base of the brain to the lower back.

Position on the feet
The reflex runs along the bony ridges from the base of the big toes to the inner ankles.

Reflexology procedure

1 Lightly run your right thumb along the bony prominence to determine the exact position of the spinal reflex.

2 Using the right thumb at an angle, caterpillar along the left reflex, from the toe to the ankle as follows:
Position a: Angle the thumb so that it is pushing up underneath the

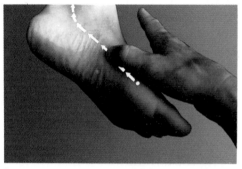

bony prominence. This is to gain access to the motor nerve reflexes which are on the abdominal side of the spine. Concentrate on this reflex when there is paralysis of movement.
Position b: Place the thumb directly onto the bony prominence to gain direct access to the vertebrae, the intervertebral discs and the spinal cord.

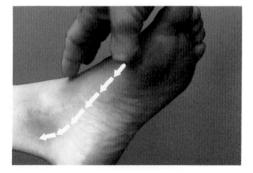

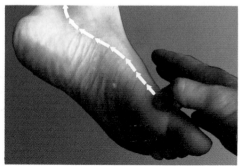

Position c: Angle the thumb so that it is pressing down on to the top of the bony ridge. This gives direct access to the sensory nerve reflexes, which are on the skin side of the spine. They should be concentrated upon when there is paralysis of sensation.

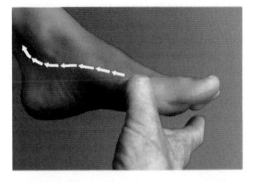

3 Massage each of these positions at least 3 times each.

4 Milk each of the 3 reflexes, from toe to ankle, at least 3 times.

5 Heal the reflexes, from toe to ankle, with light feathery movements several times.

6 Use the middle finger of the right hand to brush the surface of the skin with one stroke, from the tip of the big left toe to the ankle.

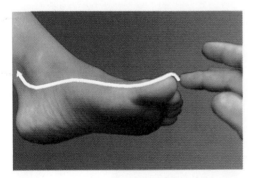

This extremely light, dynamic movement should be repeated 3 times. This particular movement unlocks past, deep rooted fears and anxieties, which are either consciously, or subconsciously, released. Each section of the spinal cord represents specific stages of foetal development, with conception being the joint on the big toe and birth the extremity below the inner ankle. The spinal cord is connected to every cell of the body through the involuntary (autonomic) nervous system.

7 Move to the right foot, keeping touch at all times, to repeat steps 1 to 6, with the left hand.

8 Having completed the massage on the right foot, hold both feet with both hands ready to relax the solar plexus reflex.

Footnote
Concentrate on the spinal reflex where congestion, gritty deposits or swelling occurs and for the following situations:

- A feeling of lack of support.
  Lack of emotional support: upper spine.
  Guilt and feeling trapped in the past: middle back.
  Deep financial concern: lower back.
  Back injury.

There will be a gap in the spinal reflex if a vertebra is missing. Curvatures or spinal abnormalities can be felt and visually detected.

The solar plexus

Position on the body
In the centre of the body immediately below the diaphragm.

Position on the foot
The solar plexus reflexes are immediately below the hard ball of the foot, stretching from the centre to the inner aspect of the foot.

Reflexology procedure

1 Place the right thumb on the left solar plexus reflex and the left thumb on the right solar plexus reflex. Keep your fingers away from the feet.

2 Check your posture. Are your shoulders, jaw and body totally relaxed? Close your eyes and breathe in deeply.

3 In this relaxed state, very gently and slowly apply pressure through both thumbs, until you feel a resistance. Stop and apply a steady pressure for a while.

4 Allow the recipient's skin to push your thumb away until you feel a pulsating sensation. This is not always obvious at first, but persevere. To find it, gently press in again and slowly release, or fractionally alter the position of your thumb. When pulsating is felt, or when your thumbs are applying minimal pressure, keep them still and relax your body for 2 to 5 minutes. Breathe deeply throughout and with each in breath imagine that you are taking in a golden liquid. As you breathe out imagine this golden liquid passing through your thumbs into the recipient. Try not to fall asleep! Sensations commonly experienced by recipients include:

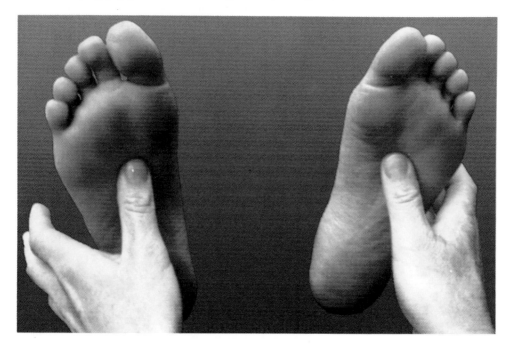

an incredible lightness or sensation of 'floating on air'

a reassuring glow below the diaphragm

'fluttering' in the abdominal region

a 'shooting' sensation followed by a wonderful release of tension

removal of a 'burden' when your thumbs draw away.

5 After 2 to 5 minutes, gently push your thumbs in again, relax and then, *very slowly* withdraw until your thumbs are hovering over the skin. Hold this position for a while as you feel a tremendous heat or vibration.

6 Immediately heal first the left reflex and then the right.

7 Hold the left foot with both hands ready to move onto the endocrine system (see page 34).

Footnote

- The solar plexus is an incredibly powerful reflex. It effectively calms and releases pent up tension. Any resistance or tightness of the reflex is indicative of extreme anxiety. Calming this reflex is particularly beneficial to those with any nervous disorders, allergies, asthma or skin irritations. It will even put young children to sleep, provided they are tired!

Maximum benefit from Reflexology is achieved through a wholistic approach, bearing the following points in mind.

- Discover peace of mind through forgiveness and a clear conscience.
- Question preconceived ideas and abandon unjustified prejudice.
- Recognise 'things of value', in the world at large, in others and in yourself, and cherish them. Finance is only necessary as a means towards independence and mobility.
- Follow 'the middle way'; extremes are never healthy.
- Be yourself. Comparison with others is fruitless for no two people are alike.
- Keep an open mind and listen, with understanding towards other points of view.
- Put quality time and energy into the here and now.
- Take control of your life. Health and happiness cannot be bought.
- Believe in yourself, after all, you are the only person you can depend upon!
- Have faith in life processes and avoid disappointment.
- Enjoy life.

The gentle Bach Flower remedies available in all health shops affect the mood and outlook and, in so doing, provide the strength to overcome draining emotions and negative states of mind. They help to maintain calmness and serenity despite tiredness, an emergency or any demanding situation.

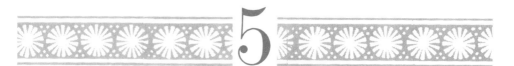
THE ENDOCRINE SYSTEM

The endocrine system detects changes inside and outside the body. It
exerts a tremendous influence over feelings and physical reactions.

Position in the body
The endocrine glands are
incredibly small, oddly shaped
pieces of tissue tucked into obscure
positions throughout the body.

Position on the feet
The miniscule reflexes of the
glands have corresponding
positions on the feet.

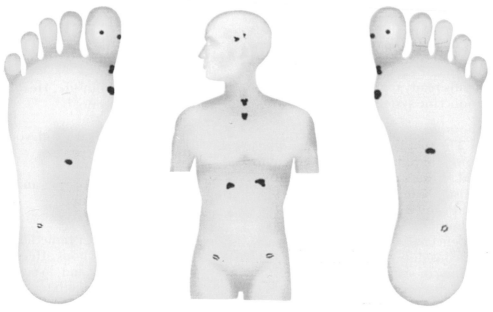

Characteristics

The endocrine glands are the chemical regulators of bodily functions,
essential for a stable internal environment. They secrete their powerful
hormones directly into the blood stream to excite or inhibit cellular
activity. In so doing, they balance and harmonise the body. Over 100
hormones are present in the blood stream at all times, although the levels
fluctuate to accommodate bodily needs. The system resembles an
orchestra, with the *pituitary gland* as the conductor. Well tuned glands
secreting the correct amount, at the right time, provide harmony.
Although each gland has a specific role to play, all are interdependent.

Effects of 'stress'

Emotional distress plays havoc with the endocrine system and imbalances the finely tuned system. Its extreme sensitivity stems from the direct influence of the *hypothalamus* in the brain. Each gland is a centre of energy, but tension deprives them of essential life forces and allows toxic wastes to block the energy flow. The distribution of hormones is affected by the reduced blood flow, whilst the vice-like grip of tension inhibits the activity of the target cells.

The endocrine system is extremely sensitive to fluctuating environmental conditions, such as weather and the body's need for sustenance, as well as emotional upsets and negative thoughts. A contented mind, with happy thoughts, has a calming, balancing effect, whilst negative emotions have detrimental effects.

Reflexology procedure

Reflexology *normalises* the workings of each gland. An overactive gland is calmed, whilst an underactive one is stimulated. Provided sensitive massage is applied it is not possible to 'overstimulate' a gland. The deep state of relaxation induced by the massage allows the free flow of blood and nutrients to both the hypothalamus and the pituitary gland, allowing both to re-establish control. If there is physical destruction of the cells, remaining cells are encouraged to function to the best of their ability, and the possibility of abnormal cells developing is reduced through the creation of a favourable environment. The massage calms the body and encourages free distribution of the hormones.

A balanced endocrine system promotes a state of balance (or 'homoeostatis') by harmonising all bodily activities and, for this reason, is massaged immediately after the central nervous system.

All the endocrine gland reflexes, with the possible exception of the pineal and thymus reflexes, are naturally sensitive, extremely so when there is an energy flow blockage.

It is important to spend time and avoid rushing when massaging these reflexes. Each reflex is massaged individually in three easy steps, first on the left foot and then on the right. Practise on your palm first to feel the effect and to achieve the most beneficial pressure. The lighter the touch, the more potent the effect.

1 Place the thumb or third finger on the reflex point and, without moving its position, apply gentle pressure and begin massaging the point with a clockwise rotation. Do this for up to a minute.

2 Keeping the thumb or finger on the reflex, stop massaging, then slowly apply gentle but firm direct pressure onto the reflex, without causing distress. Relax and allow the recipient's skin to push the digit away very slowly.

3 With both thumbs or both fingers feather stroke towards the body, barely touching the surface of the reflex point.

Footnotes

● If you are unsure of the correct reflex point, or are curious to see just how sensitive these reflexes are, place the knuckle on the reflex and push deep into the point. A word of caution: any imbalance of the gland will register in the highly sensitive reflex and the recipient may experience deep discomfort or a shooting sensation. If there is no sensation you may need to move your digit fractionally, or the angle at which you are pressing to hit the correct spot.

● Colours have a profound effect on the chemical composition of the finely tuned body. Consequently, they have a powerful impact on the body's natural healing ability.

● Clothes, food and the environment all filter colours, and provide the means by which specific colours can be used to help balance the individual endocrine glands.

The pituitary or master gland

The pituitary gland directly influences all the other glands, thereby regulating all metabolic processes.

Position in the body
The pituitary gland is a pea-sized gland at the base of the brain, immediately below the hypothalamus. It is well protected by bone and tissues.

Position on the feet
The pituitary gland reflex is halfway down the side of the big toes, behind the bony prominence which acts as a protective shield. It is a minute reflex, with half being reflected on each big toe.

Characteristics

This tiny, oval gland has two distinct parts which function independently of each other. Its body-nourishing hormone promotes growth in children and balances energy output and tissue repair in adults. Its secretions also control water balance, blood pressure and assist in uterine contraction and breast feeding after childbirth.

Psychosomatic aspect

The pituitary gland is the control centre and imbalances occur when there is loss of emotional control.

Reflexology procedure

1 Rest the left foot against the left hand. Place the ball of the right thumb below the bony prominence so that the inside edge of the thumb is in line with the top of the bony prominence.

2 Roll the edge of the thumb over the bony prominence and apply pressure in and down. You should feel a tiny swelling about the size of a pin head or smaller. If congested, it is generally taut with no definable swellings.

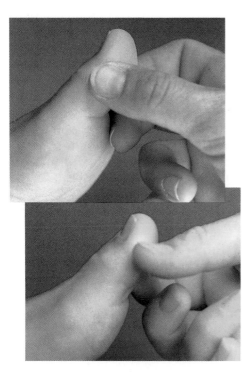

foot against the right hand. Place the left thumb on the right toe and repeat the massage on the right pituitary reflex.

7 Keep the left thumb resting against the right pituitary reflex and, at the same time, rest the right thumb against the left pituitary reflex for a few seconds, to balance the two sides of the pituitary gland.

Footnote
If there is difficulty in detecting the reflex on the right foot with the left thumb, locate it with the right thumb, but massage with the left. Concentrate on the pituitary gland for:

- Any imbalance of the endocrine system
- Metabolic disorders
- Sexual disturbances
- Growth irregularities
- Poor temperature control
- Emotional upsets
- Negativity

3 With slight pressure rotate clockwise keeping the thumb on the reflex.

4 Leave the thumb on the reflex, stop rotating and slowly apply gentle but firm pressure without causing distress. Relax and allow the recipient's skin to push the thumb away.

5 Feather stroke the area towards the body.

6 Keeping contact rest the right

The pituitary gland is more likely to remain in balance when there is control on all levels of the mind, body and spirit. A positive outlook and enjoyment of life play a vital role. Learn to cope with demands and, if necessary, review your lifestyle to eliminate irritating factors. The pituitary gland responds well to the colour indigo.

The pineal gland

The pineal gland co-ordinates biological cycles.

Position in the body
Tucked behind the pituitary gland at the base of the brain.

Position on the feet
The pineal reflex is accessed through the optic cavities found at the centre of the pads on the big

toes, where a slight hollow can be felt. (These are also the reflexes for the eye.)

Characteristics

The pineal is a tiny pine-cone-shaped gland, about half the size of the pituitary gland. Although buried in darkness, the amount of chemical substances secreted by this gland varies according to natural light fluctuations entering through the eye. Its secretion, melatonin, influences the start of sexual maturity, and helps to regulate the sexual cycle in women.

Reflexology procedure

Congestion or abnormalities of the eye reduce the amount of light entering the body, and can directly affect the functioning of the pineal gland. Massaging the optic cavity reflex re-establishes energy and blood flow, and reduces the congestion.

1 Rest the left foot against the left hand. Place the ball of the right thumb on the centre of the pad on the left big toe. As you press in gently you should feel a slight hollow beneath the surface. This is the optic cavity. It is usually in a 'bull's eye' position on the big toes.

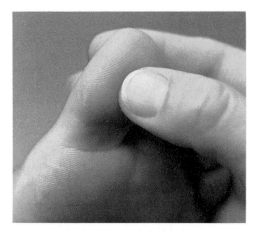

2 With a slight pressure massage the reflex with a clockwise motion.

3 Stop rotating but keep the thumb on the reflex. Slowly apply pressure without causing distress, until you meet resistance; relax and allow the recipient's skin to push the thumb away.

4 Using both fingers, feather stroke the surface in a downward movement.

5 Rest the right foot against the right hand and repeat the massage with the left thumb on the right big toe.

6 Leave the thumb resting against the right pineal reflex whilst resting the right thumb against the left pineal reflex for a while, to balance the pineal gland.

Footnote
● The recipient may feel a rotating sensation in the eye as this reflex is being massaged. Concentrate on this reflex for menstrual irregularities, especially ammenhorroea and inconsistent cycles. Women with breast cancer have been found to have reduced pineal secretions. Congestions are more likely to be related to eye disorders (see eye, page 47). The pineal responds well to violet.

The thyroid gland

The thyroid gland secretes thyroxine, a hormone which influences all the major systems of the body.

Position in the body
The thyroid gland is at the base of the throat, behind the crease in the lower neck.

Position on the feet
The thyroid gland reflex is on the lower crease at the base of both big toes. Half is found on each foot on the inner edge.

Characteristics

The thyroid is an extremely active gland with two small lobes and containing the four parathyroids. Thyroxine is essential for growth, mental alertness, digestive processes, heart function and resistance to infection.

The parathyroids regulate phosphorus and calcium levels in the blood. They control the one kilogram of calcium in the body, and store 99 percent of it in the bones. Calcium is essential for nervous functioning, blood clotting and glandular secretion.

Psychosomatic aspects

The thyroid is linked to self esteem and imbalances occur when a person feels that, in giving so much of themselves to others, they leave little or no time and energy for themselves. This causes resentment and suppressed self pity.

Underactivity   Most people suffer from a slightly underactive thyroid gland, and are afflicted with one or more of the following ailments:

Headaches; physical and emotional exhaustion; lethargy; hypoglycaemia; back pain; cramps; poor temperature control; libido loss; insomnia; depression; cholesterol imbalance; poor memory; dry, scaly skin; rigid, brittle nails; weight problems; menstrual disorders; blood pressure problems; fluid retention; a general feeling of dullness; stunted growth in children.

Although the correct amount of thyroxine may be circulating in the blood, it is of no use if, due to tension, it is not being taken up and utilised by specific target cells.

Overactive thyroid gland   Hyperthyroidism, or an overactive thyroid gland, causes extreme nervousness and an inability to relax. There is no weight gain, despite consumption of vast quantities of food, due to the high metabolic rate. Digestive disturbances, an increased heart rate and raised body temperatures further strain the body.

Overactive parathyroid glands   Too much Parathormone draws calcium from the bones, leaving them porous and brittle. The increased level of calcium in the blood increases the possibility of kidney stones.

Reflexology procedure

1 Rest the left foot against the left hand. Place the upper edge of the right thumb along the inner third of the crease at the base of the left big toe.

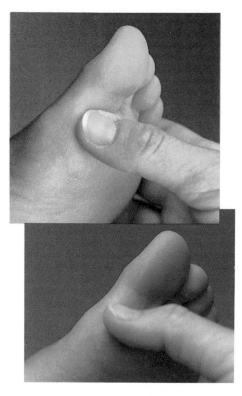

2 Roll the right thumb over the crease and then apply gentle pressure downwards to feel for a tiny distinctive swelling tucked behind the crease. If congested there will be a tenseness in the area.

3 Once the reflex has been located, massage in a clockwise rotation.

4 Gently press down onto the reflex, without distressing the recipient, until you feel resistance, relax and allow your thumb to be pushed away.

5 Using two digits brush the surface of the reflex with feather-like, downward strokes.

6 Rest the right foot against the right hand, and repeat the massage. If you have difficulty detecting the reflex with your left hand, find it with your right thumb but massage with your left thumb.

7 Keep the left thumb resting against the right thyroid reflex and, at the same time, place the right thumb against the left reflex. Hold for a few seconds to balance the thyroid gland.

Footnotes
● The reflex will feel swollen, gritty or extremely tense when there is an energy flow blockage. Concentrate on this reflex if the person is complaining of metabolic disorders, general exhaustion, insomnia, headaches, sexual disturbances, muscle rigidity, extreme irritability or excitability, growth retardation or any of the ailments mentioned above. Post menopausal women are prone to brittle bones so stimulate this gland particularly in women over the age of 30. The thyroid gland responds well to turquoise.
● If you suspect hypothyroidism, consult a naturopathic or homoeopathic doctor regarding natural thyroxine supplements.
● Regular Reflexology will normalise the action over a period of time.
● Make time for yourself, to be yourself and do what you would like to do. Release your creativity through the free expression of your needs.

The thymus gland

The thymus gland actively directs all the immune forces within the body, particularly at times when the body is most vulnerable to disease – in the very young and the elderly.

Position in the body
The thymus gland rests against the breast bone, just below the thyroid gland, in a small indentation where the two clavicle bones meet.

Position on the feet
The thymus gland reflex is situated on the sole of the feet, approximately halfway down the ball, against the inner aspect.

Characteristics

The pinkish-grey thymus gland shields most of the breast bone at birth and doubles in size by the age of 12. It then shrivels and remains calcified for the greater span of life, until it grows again later in life, when it is believed to play a vital role in the ageing process.

Thymosin, the secretion from the thymus gland, helps to convert white blood cells into 'killer' T-cells, which attack certain bacteria, cancer cells, fungi, viruses and other harmful substances. Thymus cells migrate to other parts of the body to become centres of lymphatic activity. The *Peyer's Patches*, small collections of lymph nodes within the small intestine, are of particular importance since there is a correlation between a reduced number of patches and a weakened body.

Warriors and gorillas instinctively beat their chests before going into battle or a fight to stimulate the thymus gland and build up the immune forces in case of injury!

Underactivity   An underactive thymus gland immediately reduces the immune system making the body more vulnerable to disease and infection, especially during periods of distress and depression.

AIDS and myalgic encephalomyelitis sufferers have lowered immunity with little or no activity of the thymus gland. Myalgic encephalomyelitis, otherwise known as 'Yuppie Flu', occurs when persistent viral infections attack the muscles, brain and central nervous system.

Overactivity   Increased thymus secretions create an overactive immune system which, in extreme cases, can lead to self destruction.

Psychosomatic implications

An imbalanced thymus gland indicates extreme vulnerability and hyper-sensitivity. It is accompanied by the belief that all actions, belief systems and expressions of individuality are under attack. AIDS and myalgic encelphalomyelitis sufferers believe that they are being persecuted by the world and they have no faith in their self worth. AIDS victims are often besieged by sexual guilt.

Reflexology procedure

1 Place the right thumb or third finger on the slight depression halfway down the inner edge of the ball of the left foot, directly below the thyroid gland.

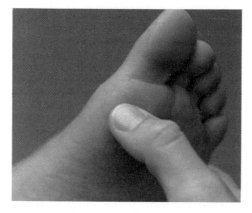

2 Gently massage the reflex with a clockwise motion.

3 Keep the finger on the reflex as you stop rotating, gently press the area, relax and allow the recipient's skin to push the thumb or finger away.

4 Heal the area stroking downwards towards the heel.

5 Repeat the massage with the left thumb on the right thyroid reflex.

6 Leave the left thumb resting against the right thymus gland reflex and, at the same time, rest the right thumb against the left thymus gland reflex for a few seconds, to balance the two sides of the thymus gland.

Footnotes
- This reflex is particularly important in babies, young children and the elderly. Concentrate on the thymus reflex during the winter season. It is generally very sensitive and needs extra attention when the body is fighting an infection, HIV or mylagic encelphalomyelitis.
- To re-establish a strong immune system it is important to feel confident and comfortable with your own beliefs. Love yourself so that others can grow to love you. Learn to feel safe in the world and amongst its people. The thymus gland responds well to green.

The adrenal glands

The adrenal glands play a major role in preparing the body for emergencies. They also control inflammatory conditions as well as the salt and water balance in the body.

Position in the body
The adrenal glands crown the kidneys and are found towards the back of the abdominal cavity. The right adrenal glad is slightly lower and a little more central than the left, due to the bulk of the liver being on the right side of the body.

Position on the feet
The adrenal gland reflexes are immediately below the solar plexus reflex, with the right gland being fractionally lower and slightly more central.

Characteristics

There are at least 30 steroid hormones secreted by the adrenal glands.
The right gland is pyramidal in shape while the left gland is semi-lunar.
Each gland has two distinct parts, an outer cortex and an extremely
vascular internal medulla, which receive a rich supply of sympathetic
nerves from the coelic plexus.

The cortex secretes steroids which regulate electrolyte metabolism,
maintain a stable watery environment, assist with carbohydrate
metabolism, influence the blood sugar level, combat inflammation and
allergies, and influence the development and functioning of the
reproductive organs which determine the physical and temperamental
characteristics of the male and female.

Adrenaline and noradrenaline, the two secretions from the medulla,
trigger a set of similar responses in the sympathetic nervous system,
which prepare the body for 'fight and flight'. Adrenaline immediately
responds to physiological and psychological 'stress', with an instant surge
of fuel from the liver providing super human strength as the body is
alerted for an emergency.

Underactivity   Rheumatoid arthritis, allergies and other inflammatory
conditions are more likely to occur with reduced levels of cortisone. A
constant lack of energy with reduced blood sugar levels and gastro-
intestinal upsets can lead to excessive weight loss.

Overactivity   Cortisol levels increase tenfold to combat 'stress'. If the
high levels continue there is lowered resistance to disease.

Effects of 'stress'

When the body is distressed it is alerted into a defensive mode with an
outpouring of adrenaline – a mechanism reserved for emergency
situations only. However, there is usually a consistently high level of
adrenaline in the blood, due to the ever present emotional, physical and
environmental factors which surround and constantly alarm the body.
Muscles are permanently tense, the heart overworks, energy is burnt up
too quickly until eventually the whole system is exhausted. When an
emergency situation does arise, the body and mind are not able to cope.
The anti-inflammatory effect minimises the sensation of pain and often
temporarily masks the severity of symptoms. Signs of extreme distress
are often referred to as 'burn-out'.

Psychosomatic implications

Imbalances of the adrenal glands are more likely when there is a feeling
of hopelessness, anxiety and defeatism. A feeling of inadequacy may
make the person feel like giving up the fight.

Reflexology procedure

1 Place the right thumb on the left foot immediately below the solar plexus reflex. Feel for a distinctive swelling below the skin's surface. It may be fractionally lower or slightly more central in some people. If you have difficulty, alter the angle of the thumb to redistribute the pressure.

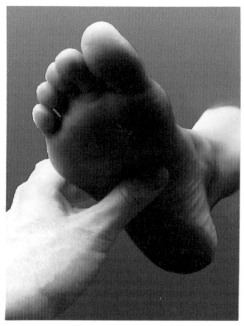

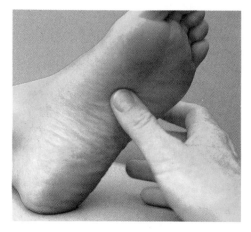

2 Gently rotate the thumb in a clockwise motion for at least a minute.

3 Keep the thumb on the reflex as you stop rotating, gently apply pressure, relax and allow the recipient's skin to push the thumb away.

4 Heal the area by gently stroking downwards, towards the heel.

5 Repeat the procedure with the left thumb on the right adrenal reflex, which is slightly lower and more central. Again feel for a deep swelling.

6 Keep the left thumb resting on the right adrenal reflex whilst resting the right thumb on the left adrenal reflex, for a few seconds, to balance the two adrenal glands.

Footnotes
● If there is an energy flow blockage there may be a tiny 'water bubble' or gritty deposits on the reflex. An imbalanced adrenal reflex is extremely sensitive, and there may be an uncomfortable 'bruising' sensation if excessive pressure is applied.
● A more sensitive and prolonged massage is required for all nervous disorders, 'burn out', allergies (including asthma), inflammatory conditions from boils to arthritis, water and mineral imbalances such as oedema and urinary problems, sexual disorders, all menstrual related conditions, hypoglycaemia, irregular blood pressure, heart strain, muscular tension, and lowered resistance to disease.
● Self-approval builds confidence and self esteem necessary for the recognition of self worth. The adrenal glands respond well to orange.

Pancreas

The pancreas is an endocrine and an exocrine gland. Both of its functions are linked to the digestive process and so, for the purpose of Reflexology, it is massaged with the digestive tract. (See page 73.)

Gonadotrophic or sex hormones

MALE: The testes secrete testerone which determines the male characteristics. FEMALE: The ovaries produce oestrogen and progesterone responsible for the development of female characteristics and function of the reproductive organs. The menstrual cycle depends on these hormones. (See reproductive system page 94.)

Position in the body
Male   The male reproductive glands, the testes, are suspended in the scrotum. The prostate gland surrounds the neck of the bladder and part of the ureter.
Female   The female reproductive glands are in the lesser pelvis, either side of the uterus.

Position on the feet
Male   The testes and prostate reflexes are both reflected onto the inner aspect of the feet, near the base of the heel and midway between the ankle and heel respectively.
Female   The ovary reflexes can be approached from two directions.
a   On the sole of the feet in the extreme lower corners in the fleshy hollows, towards the outer edge of the feet.
b   On the outer heel – midway between the tip of the heel and ankle bone.

Characteristics

Male   Each testis is ovoid with a crescent shaped, highly coiled tube behind it called the epididymis. The prostate consists of gland tissue surrounded by plain muscle.
Female   The ovaries resemble an almond both in shape and size. They are filled with immature female germ cells and mature ova and secrete six different oestrogens.

Imbalance of the sex glands   Undersecretion of sex hormones during puberty can prevent full development of secondary sex characteristics. A decrease or absence of the female hormones results in ammenhorroea (no menstrual cycle), and possible infertility.

Psychosomatic implications

Imbalances of the sexual glands are generally guilt related, or stem from the belief that sex is sinful or 'dirty'. Subconsciously it can create a physical barrier if there is anger towards the spouse or a parent. Sexual pressures clamp down on the free flow of these hormones.

Reflexology procedure

Females only:

1 Place the right thumb on the left foot where the hard skin of the outer edge of the ball of the foot forms an inverted 'L'. This is the ovary reflex.

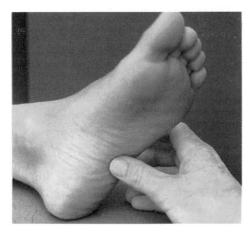

2 Massage in a clockwise motion.

3 As you stop massaging apply gentle pressure and push into the reflex. Relax and allow the recipient's skin to push the thumb away.

4 Gently heal with light downward strokes.

5 Repeat the massage on the right foot with the left thumb.

6 Leave the left thumb resting against the right ovary reflex and, at the same time, rest the right thumb against the left ovary reflex for a few seconds, to balance the two ovaries.

Footnote

● Massage the ovaries even if they have been removed to stimulate any remaining tissue that may regenerate in favourable circumstances. Each month the ovaries take turns to ovulate. The active ovary is always more swollen and sensitive. The contraceptive pill suppresses ovulation and generally reduces sensitivity making it difficult to detect the ovarian reflexes.

Males and females:

1 Place the right third finger midway between the heel and ankle on the outer aspect of the left foot where there is a slight indentation. This reflex is the secondary access to the ovaries but since it is also the reflex for the high stress area situated in the hollow above the buttocks it is also massaged in males.

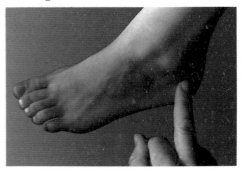

2 Gently rotate clockwise.

3 As you stop, gently press into the reflex, relax and allow the recipient's skin to push the finger away.

4 Gently heal with light upward stroking movements.

5 Repeat on the right foot with the left middle finger.

6 Rest the left finger on the right reflex and the right finger on the left reflex for a while, to balance these reflexes.

The prostate (male) reflex and vaginal (female) reflex

1 Place the left thumb or middle finger on the visible hollow midway between the heel and ankle on the inner aspect of the left foot.

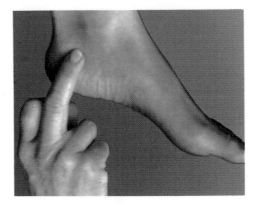

2 Repeat the massage on both feet.

3 Balance by resting the left thumb on the right reflex and the right thumb on the left reflex.

The testes (male) and pubic bone (female) reflexes

1 Place the left thumb or third finger on the back of the ankle, just above the heel.

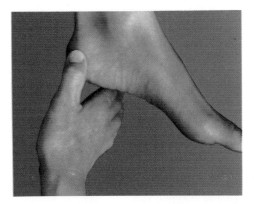

2 Massage as above on both feet.

3 Leave the left finger resting on the right reflex whilst resting the right thumb against the left reflex for a few seconds, to balance the reflexes.

Footnotes
● Concentrate on the sex glands in young children, during puberty and adolescence, during pregnancy, and for menstrual disorders. The sex glands respond well to red.
● Feel comfortable with your sexuality and enjoy the pleasures of receiving from, and giving love to, the special person in your life.
● Having calmed the nervous system and also the endocrine system it is now possible to proceed with the rest of the massage.

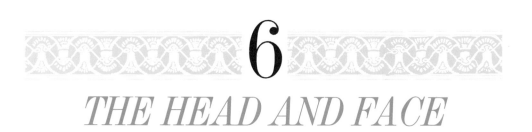

6
THE HEAD AND FACE

The head is an amazing extension of the body from which all the bodily processes are monitored and detected. It stores the remarkable intellectual centre and sensory devices.

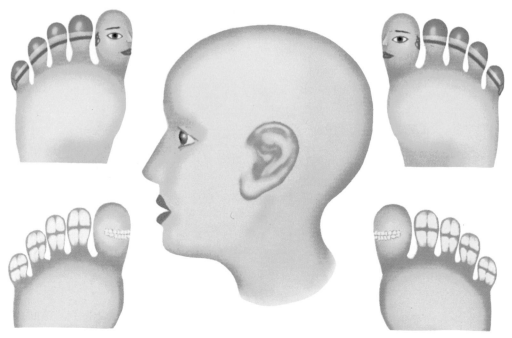

Characteristics

The sensory organs pour vivid reports into the brain, providing vital information for analysis, which is then acted upon by the rest of the body. There is constant communication and awareness between the cells in the body and those in the head. The face reflects fluctuating moods and feelings, although many people have learnt to mask their true emotions.

Effects of 'stress'

Blood flows against gravity to reach the extremities of the head and is immediately affected by tension which contracts muscles, inhibits blood flow and subsequently reduces the supply of vital forces. Toxic substances accumulate resulting in headaches, migraines, eye strain, hearing impairments, sinus problems and tooth decay.

Reflexology procedure

Reflexology effectively relaxes the muscles, re-establishes a healthy blood flow and allows the cells to function effectively and normally.

The eyes

The eyes are highly specialised sensory organs which alter light into an enormous wealth of bright and colourful meaningful images from which information can be gleaned and danger can be detected. They absorb 85 percent of life's experience thereby affecting the course of events. The absorbed light fills the body with light and vibrancy which impregnates every cell with energy and vitality.

Position in the body
Within the orbits of the skull.

Position on the feet
The main reflex is in the centre of the pad on the big toe, where a slight indentation can be felt. Other reflexes are in the centre of the pads on the little toes.

Characteristics

The eyes are phenomenal projections of brain tissue which come to the surface to meet the outside world. They are highly accurate, versatile and self repairing, demanding little or no attention from the user, as they happily accommodate themselves to bodily needs.

There are 28,000 nerve fibres in the eyes which instinctively adapt to the fluctuating intensity of light. The eyes speak the language of iridology through microscopic symbolic reflections on the iris which indicate the constitutional health of specific organs.

Nurturing the eyes   All essential nutrients are provided by the extensive blood supply and by tears. Blinking cleanses the eye, destroys bacteria and determines the speed at which the eyes are nurtured. The eye requires natural sunlight and certain vitamins and minerals to enhance bodily growth and vitality, and for calming the nervous system. Constant movement and stimulation is essential for keeping the eye muscles elastic and versatile.

Effect of 'stress'

Over 60 percent of people in the Western world rely on artificial devices and an increasing number experience eye strain and reduced visual perception. The degree of anxiety experienced when eyes are being tested tends to reduce visual capacity, resulting in prescribed aids being too strong for everyday use. The eyes weaken as they adapt to cope. If the lens prescription is reduced to around 83.5 percent the eyes strengthen and vision improves, until eventually they can be weaned off any form of visual aid. (*Seeing beyond 20/20* by Dr Robert Michael Kaplan O.D. M.Ed.)

Fluorescent and electric lights, windscreens spectacles and windows deprive the eyes of contact with the natural sunlight, upsetting the delicate balance of the nervous system and causing eyestrain. Staring at computers, television, books and fine intricate work deprives the eyes of oxygen and nourishment, as blinking virtually stops and breathing becomes almost negligible, thus reducing optimum performance.

The degree to which certain foods, such as simple, refined sugars and dairy products adversely effect and weaken the eyes varies from one individual to another.

Psychosomatic aspects

The eyes radiate and reveal the inner-being, personality and emotional state. (See *Iridology* by Farida Sharon MD (MA) MH ND FBRI.) Two way communication can be inhibited by shyness, anger, greed, fear, unhappiness, lack of interest, selfishness. Eyes speak volumes without a word being spoken. Children enthusiastically seek interaction with the world with wide eyes but often learn to avoid direct eye contact because of fear and shyness.

The eyes represent the ability to see all aspects of life – past, present and future. The present state of the eyes reflect past emotions, thoughts, angers, fears and beliefs which can impair visual perception. When upsetting past experiences are blocked out for fear of having to re-live the terrifying event, tension occurs which constricts the muscles and reduces the mobility of the eyes.

Near-sightedness often occurs within 18 months to 2 years of a traumatic experience, due to a blinding fear of having to look too far ahead into the future. Far-sightedness, common amongst the elderly, arises from the tendency to plan continually for the future and look ahead. It can be brought about through anger either at the self or towards other people; accompanied by the urge to be independent and to pull away from the present situation. Lazy eyes avoid the need to embrace the realities and facts of life.

Fear, anxiety and anger temporarily impede the clarity of sight, and people often turn a 'blind eye'. Night-blindness results from a deep-seated fear of the dark.

Children often develop eye problems to avoid seeing what is going on in their life, especially within the family unit. This is particularly common after a traumatic divorce.

Reflexology procedure

This is the same as for the pineal gland. (See page 36 and also pages 51–52, massage for the sinus, teeth, ear and eye reflexes.)

Footnotes
- Eye strain and visual disturbances inhibit the free flow of energy and the reflex will either be tense and bulging, or soft and spongy. Concentrate on this reflex for any eye problem and on people who work with computers or rely on visual aids.
- Exercise the eyes regularly by keeping your head still, breathing deeply and moving the eyes from one extremity to another in all directions, for example, from the extreme right to the extreme left.
- Consciously blink frequently, particularly when working on a computer, watching television or performing intricate tasks.
- Nurture the eyes by providing them with essential nutrients through a balanced diet.
- Take time to breathe in large quantities of air.
- Appreciate your sight for it is so often taken for granted.
- When you **look** make sure you **see** by observing all the small details and wondrous facets of life.

The ears

The ears are sensory structures that convert environmental sound waves into nervous impulses for interpretation by the brain. In so doing, they affect physical and emotional development. They also provide the senses of hearing, posture and balance, and are of primary importance in the formation of speech.

Position in the body
The ears are extensions on the side of the head.

Position on the feet
The inner ear reflex is midway down the inside of the big toe where there is a slight indentation. The middle ear reflexes run horizontally through the centre of each little toe to their outer edge where the outer ear reflexes are situated.

Characteristics

Vibrational frequencies of between 16 and 40,000 per second can be detected and interpreted as sound. The brain must have had previous exposure to a sound in order to understand and interpret it. A foreign language, for example, can be heard but not necessarily understood. Hearing, essential for the development of speech and a means of verbal communication, is the basis for healthy human relationships.

Effects of 'stress'

Tension has a detrimental effect on the organs of hearing, balance and posture. Muscles constrict and deprive the cells of essential life forces, causing poor cell functioning and formation. Stagnation of the vital processes dampens the clarity and acuteness of hearing. Sensitivity to lower sounds remain throughout life, but there can be a rapid decline in the degree of sensitivity to higher sounds after adolescence.

Negative, cluttered thoughts crowd the mind and can block the hearing process. Emotional distress distorts and amplifies the meaning and interpretation of words, aggravating the situation.

Loud noises have a greater wave amplitude than soft sounds and if strong enough can cause pain or damage. Highly amplified waves, such as disco music, are a cause for concern.

Lowered immunity opens the channels to the invasion of bacteria and viruses from respiratory tract infections. Children are particularly vulnerable because their eustachian tubes are shorter and narrower, and their adenoids are larger.

Psychosomatic implications

The ears represent the ability to hear and absorb what is being said. Music, words and sounds have an immediate impact on the body and emotions. The brain's interpretation can excite happiness or anger, soothe, irritate, or stir past memories. This immediately affects the state of muscles and bodily systems. Earache, particularly common in youngsters, is often a self protective device to avoid hearing verbal, or even non-verbal, parental conflict. It is possible to be conveniently deaf or intentionally to misinterpret what is being heard to avoid internal conflict. Deafness can arise from a feeling of rejection or persistent stubbornness, and acts as a means of total isolation. It may result from irrational blocking out of other opinions and ideas.

Reflexology procedure

1 Place the right middle finger on the small depression halfway down the left big toe and gently rotate with a clockwise motion.

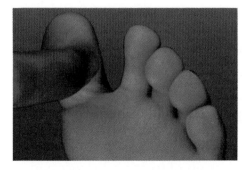

2 Keep the finger on the reflex as you stop rotating, gently apply a firm pressure, relax and allow the recipient's skin to push the thumb away.

3 Feather stroke downwards.

4 Place your left middle finger on the right inner ear reflex and repeat the massage.

Footnote
• The inner ear reflex can be extremely sensitive and needs to be massaged gently. The reflexes on the little toes are massaged with the sinus and teeth reflexes (see pages 51–52). Concentrate on this reflex for any hearing, postural or balance disorders, for dizziness and tinnitus (ringing in the ears).

The sinuses

The sinuses reduce the weight of the cranium and assist in balancing the heavy skull on the light neck. The sinuses give the voice its resonance and broaden the range of the speaker's voice.

Position in the body
There are eight nasal sinuses in the head. One pair immediately above the eyebrows; a second pair either side of the bridge of the nose; a third pair behind the nose and, the largest and most commonly known, in the cheekbones.

Position on the feet
The main access to the sinus reflexes is across the tips of the little toes, although they are also present in the central section of the big toe.

Characteristics

The sinuses are hollow air-filled cavities connected to the nasal passages and lined with tiny hairs and a mucous membrane.

Effects of 'stress'

The connection with the nasal passages makes the sinuses vulnerable to inhaled foreign particles such as dust and pollen. The irritated mucous linings swell and impinge on the nerve endings resulting in extreme discomfort which is interpreted as congestion, headaches or migraines. The voice becomes nasal as there are no spaces in which it can resound. If the mucous lining becomes infected, sinusitis occurs. Sneezing is a reflex action to dislodge and expel foreign matter from the congested passages. Distress lowers the body's immunity and increases its vulnerability to allergic and irritant factors.

Psychosomatic disorders

Those who are constantly irritated by people, situations and events are prone to sinus imbalances. Hayfever indicates congested emotions and a subconscious awareness of spring, indicated by its seasonal nature.

Reflexology procedure

The sinus reflexes are massaged with the teeth reflexes (see pages 52–53). The drainage of the little toes towards the big toe is extremely effective in flushing out the sinuses with an immediate reflex action accompanied by an outpouring of mucus. This trickles down the back of the throat causing coughing or swallowing. Areas of congestion can be pinpointed on the toes. The little toe represents the outer cheek, whilst the second toe reflects the area next to the nasal passages. The lymphatic reflexes down the sides of the toes should be massaged thoroughly to drain away the excessive mucus discharge.

Footnote
Avoid cigarette smoke and certain foods, such as dairy products and wines which irritate the mucous lining and produce more secretions in an attempt to flush out the toxins. Drink plenty of purified water throughout the day. Tolerate other people's 'peculiarities', and avoid being irritated by trivia.

The teeth

The teeth bite, chew food and are actively involved in speech. They can be aesthetically pleasing!

Position in the body
Embedded in the gums and jaw sockets.

Position on the feet
Each little toe represents two teeth up and two teeth down, with the wisdom teeth on the little toes and the incisors on the second toe – a total of 32! Small children only display 20 milk teeth initially.

Effects of 'stress'

The teeth are prone to decay due to the presence of bacteria and the diminished blood supply through 'stress'. Acid from the dental plaque erodes the enamel, destroys the dentine and inflames the pulp, which can lead to the formation of an abscess. Discolouration, the brown staining on the surface of the teeth, may be due to nicotine, the result of certain drugs, such as tetracycline, or the after affects of a severe attack of childhood illness. Deficiency of calcium and vitamin D weakens the teeth, particularly during pregnancy when the fetus draws on the mother's supplies. Nine out of ten adults suffer from a mild form of swollen, bleeding gums, known as gingivitis, at some stage of their life with pregnant women and diabetics being particularly susceptible.

Psychosomatic disorders

Teeth represent the decision to take in new ideas and food for thought. Tooth disorders indicate long term dilemmas and indecisiveness. Ideas cannot be broken down sufficiently for analysis by the brain, preventing a decision from being made. Halitosis, bad breath, stems from deep rooted anger, dissatisfaction, vile thoughts, vindictive attitudes and foul gossip.

Reflexology procedure

For sinus, teeth, ear and eye reflexes

1 Support the left toes with your left hand.

2 Caterpillar in vertical strips, with your right thumb, down each toe, thoroughly massaging the pad of each toe, starting on the outside of the little toe. Work each strip at least 3 to 4 times.

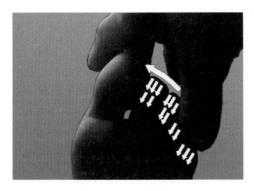

3 Milk the strips, 2 to 3 times each down the individual toes, making sure that you include the sides as you move from lesser to greater.

4 Feather stroke with light downward movements using both hands.

5 Support the toes of the right foot with the right hand and repeat the massage with the left thumb.

The throat

The throat channels vital components from the environment into the body. It is the avenue of vocal expression and creativity.

Position in the body
At the front of the neck between the chin and collar bone.

Position on the feet
The reflex is across the neck of all the toes, particularly the big toe.

Effects of 'stress'

Tension lowers the immune system, opening the way for the invasion of foreign substances, symptomised as the common sore throat, pharyngitis or laryngitis. The latter is often accompanied by the loss of voice.

Psychosomatic implications

If either expression or creativity is stifled through fear, anger or stubbornness, the person can become choked with emotion. The restrictions imposed by society are largely responsible for inhibiting expression of feelings, ideas and thoughts, causing words to be swallowed or stilled. People fear ridicule, are sensitive to the feelings of others, or are concerned for the consequences. Young children frequently complain of sore throats, indicating frustration at not being allowed or being capable of expressing their true emotions. Post nasal drip (the trickling of mucus down the back of the throat) occurs when the person is feeling victimised and can be a form of internal crying. It generally occurs during and after traumatic emotional events.

Reflexology procedure

1 Gently hold the left toes back with the left hand.

2 Using the right thumb caterpillar down the necks of each toe, 3 to 4 times, starting on the little toe and working inwards.

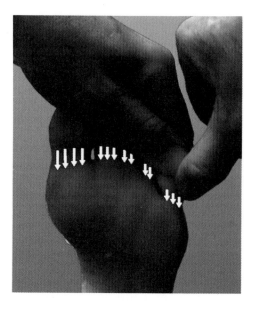

3 Concentrate on the neck of the big toe, the main throat reflex, and massage an extra few times.

4 Milk the toes thoroughly, especially down the sides.

5 Heal the area gently with tiny downward strokes using two digits.

6 Repeat the massage on the right foot with the right hand holding the toes back as you massage with the left thumb.

Footnote
● Concentrate on the throat when there is an infection or post nasal drip, and particularly during winter.

The face

The face provides a protective shield to the vital sensory and intellectual apparatus, and is a portal for all energising life forces. Facial expressions reflect innermost emotions and thoughts.

Position in the body
The front of the head from the temple to the jawline.

Position on the feet
The face is mainly reflected onto the ball of the big toes.

Characteristics

The face is generally the most exposed part of the body. Young children openly express themselves through their faces, but learn to control their expressions as they grow older as they are expected to conform to social expectations.

Effects of 'stress'

Worry lines indicate long term anxieties. Extreme tension, anger, resentment and a need for revenge cause the jaws to clench unconsciously with pain extending from the face to the neck and shoulders. Ringing in the ears, slight loss of hearing, blurred vision, clicking jaws and clenched teeth are all characteristic symptoms of this common disorder. Acne is exacerbated by social, parental and school pressures, poor eating habits, insufficient sleep, little or no exercise and a sluggish excretory system. Teenage boys are often victims due to increased activity of sex hormones.

Hair immediately reflects tension, exhaustion, detrimental effects of drugs, nutritional and hormonal imbalances.

Psychosomatic implications

The face reflects our innermost thoughts and feelings. Poor skin indicates a poor self image and a need to barricade the self against the outside world.

Reflexology procedure

The face is massaged at the same time as the brain reflex on the big toe (see pages 25–26).

Footnotes

- Concentrate on the tip of the big toe, over the temple reflex for headaches and migraines, and along the lower part of the pad, over the jaw reflex.
- Learn to relax shoulders, neck and jawline, breathing deeply at the same time. Consciously do this when feeling uptight, driving or when in a challenging situation. Passively mobilise and exercise the relaxed jaw.
- Fill your mind with positive thoughts and find inner peace.

For acne

- Regular Reflexology reduces the enormity of parental, school and social pressures and provides the strength to cope.
- Eat fresh fruits and vegetables rather than unnatural and refined products.
- Enjoy a good night's sleep every night and find time to relax totally, breathe deeply and reflect.
- Adopt an intensive skin cleaning programme and include regular facials.
- Make time to exercise, preferably outside.
- Enjoy life and make the most of your health and vitality.

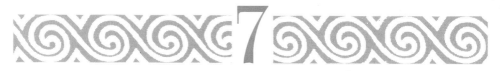

7

THE LYMPHATIC SYSTEM

Like an extensive sewerage network, the lymphatic system neutralises and flushes out harmful substances to clean the body and makes space for fresh supplies of essential life forces.

Position in the body
Lymphatic tissue is present throughout the body, with the exception of the brain, bone, cartilage and teeth, but is concentrated in particular sites.

Position on the feet
The lymphatic reflexes are present throughout the foot, with corresponding concentrations.

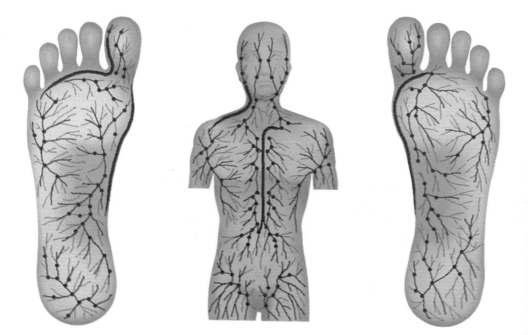

Characteristics

The lymphatic system forms a vast interlinked network with the circulatory system to drain away excess fluid, unwanted wastes and toxins. Extremely fine open-ended lymphatic capillaries are superficially scattered throughout the body, and join together to form larger collapsible vessels.

Strategically placed along these vessels are over 100 minute oval shaped swellings (nodes) which contain fibrous traps to purify the lymph and prevent the spread of infection. They are concentrated in the throat, armpits and groins and swell considerably during an infection to combat invading particles. The vessels join to form lymphatic ducts which return the fresh lymph to the blood stream in the shoulder region. The lymph is moved against gravity by respiratory motion and muscular activity.

By keeping the fluid level balanced, cells are prevented from swelling and becoming distorted. Lymph plays a vital role in the defence mechanism and is vital for absorption and distribution of fats from the small intestine.

Effects of 'stress'

Tension disrupts the rhythmic, smooth flow of lymph causing a backlog which impedes the drainage of toxic wastes from the tissues. The build-up of poisons burden the body and drain it of its vitality. Oedema, swelling of the extremities, is indicative of this condition.

Psychosomatic implications

Problems with the lymphatics serve as a warning that the mind has become so obstructed by draining negative forces that the healthy flow of life's forces has become blocked.

Reflexology procedure

The lymphatic system is continually drained throughout Reflexology massage, although there are particular areas that require specific attention at various stages of the massage (see also pages 87–88). The first lymphatics to be milked are either side of each toe, representing the concentration of lymphatic tissue on either side of the face.

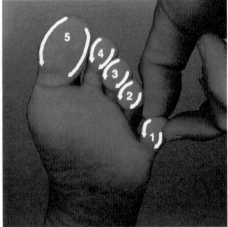

1 Support the left little toe between the left forefinger and thumb.

2 Gently squeeze down either side of the toe from top to bottom, between the right thumb and finger.

3 Repeat the milking on every toe.

4 Support the right little toe with the right hand fingers and squeeze either side of each toe with the left thumb and finger.

The second reflex to be massaged is found along the narrow strip immediately below the small toes as far as the big toe, which is set lower than the other toes. The lymphatic ducts pour their contents back into the blood in this region.

1 Gently hold back the little toes on the left foot with the left hand.

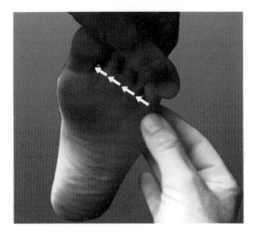

2 Caterpillar horizontally along the base of the toes with the right thumb from lesser to greater. Repeat a few times.

3 This is the only time that milking is across the foot. Wastes are then ready to be channelled through the toes at a later stage. Using the right thumb gently milk the reflex from lesser to greater a few times.

4 Heal the area with light downward feather movements.

5 Repeat all the steps on the right foot with the left thumb.

Footnote
● These lymphatic reflexes will feel taut when there are ear, eye or nose congestions.

8

THE THORACIC REGION

Position in the body
The upper part of the thoracic torso is relatively immobile, mimicking the rigidity of the skull whilst the ribs are relatively free, like the limbs. It houses most of the respiratory tract and the heart, part of the digestive tract and a complex network of blood, nerves and lymphatic vessels, all of which are well protected by skin, bone and muscles.

Position on the feet
The thoracic region is reflected onto the balls of the feet, immediately below the necks of the toes.

The respiratory system

Breath is the very essence of life and the respiratory process allows for the gaseous exchange between the body and its environment.

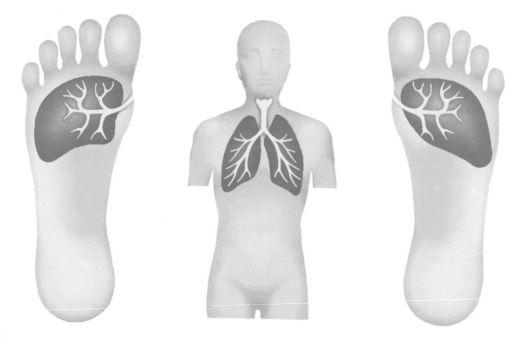

Position in the body
Extends from the nose through the throat to occupy most of the thoracic cavity.

Position on the feet
The reflex runs down the inner aspect of each foot from the middle of the big toe and occupies the balls of both feet.

Characteristics

The ribcage has an amazing capacity for expansion and contraction as the breath of life is inhaled and bodily wastes are exhaled, either consciously or unconsciously. The balance of acceptance and rejection is vital to health. Oxygen is the combustible element which allows the release of energy, as the breath circulates the body 360 times, whilst carbon dioxide is a poisonous waste product.

The body gives high priority to the involuntary task of breathing. The build-up of internal pollution (carbon dioxide), rather than the lack of essential supplies (oxygen), triggers the respiratory centres in the brain.

The diaphragm, a strong dome-shaped sheet of skeletal muscle, separates the thoracic cavity from the abdominal cavity and plays an active role in respiration, sneezing, coughing, sighing, crying and hiccups.

Effects of 'stress'

Breath is restrained to suppress disturbing emotions and during periods of intense concentration. Distress immediately disrupts the rhythmic pattern of expansion and contraction, depriving the body of oxygen. If this state is prolonged, cells will shrival or malfunction with the possibility of abnormal cell growth as in cancer.

Rapid breathing, known as hyperventilation, is due to extreme anxiety. Too much carbon dioxide is expelled, upsetting the gaseous balance. It can be eased by cupping the hands over the nose and mouth so that the carbon dioxide is inhaled back into the body until the balance has been restored.

Lowered immunity opens the respiratory tract to attack by airborne bacteria and viruses. The common cold, caused by 200 or so viruses, often leads to respiratory tract infection, of which bronchitis and pneumonia are the more serious.

Irritating or emotional factors throw the bronchi into spasm. Irritants are removed from the nasal mucosa through sneezing, and from the airways through coughing.

Psychosomatic implications

Breathing represents the ability to take in lungfulls of life forces. Breathing problems indicate a poor self image leading to a deprivation of life's breaths. Children who are smothered in love by a parent or relation may become anxious about breathing on their own or may feel so stifled that they panic, resulting in bronchial spasm, known as asthma. Asthmatic attacks can also be a form of suppressed crying. Belief that it is hereditary arises from similar attitudes being handed down from generation to generation.

Bronchitis arises from an inflamed environment in the home or at the place of work, where there is constant bickering, shouting and arguing, or where anger is being suppressed by stony silence. Pneumonia sufferers seem to carry emotional scars and often become disillusioned with life. Emphysema sufferers generally feel unworthy or too frightened to take in all that life offers. Hyperventilation occurs when there is an acute fear of the future, and is a defence mechanism to resist change.

The power of Reflexology

The art of breathing does not need to be taught but liberated. Reflexology releases the tension from the postural muscles and provides the whole body with a greater supply of oxygen. Each cell can then receive its required quota of energy and oxygen and be kept clean of toxic gases.

Deep expiration causes the pelvis to roll forward and releases pent-up sexual tension. Breasts are firmed by the good supply of blood which irrigates the whole organism.

Reflexology procedure

The air passage reflexes were massaged with the face and throat reflexes and so it is only necessary to massage the chest reflex at this stage.

2 Caterpillar in vertical strips with the right thumb from beneath the little toe to the diaphragm reflex. Repeat 3 to 4 times.

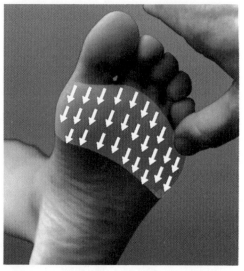

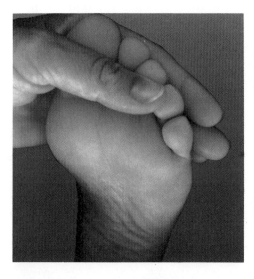

1 Rest the upper half of the left foot against the open left hand.

3 Continue to caterpillar in vertical strips, 3 to 4 times each, from lesser to greater, across the ball of the foot as far as the inside of the foot.

4 Milk down the same strips 3 to 4 times each with both thumbs, from lesser to greater.

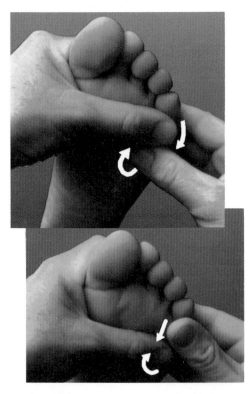

5 Place the knuckle of the right third finger at the top of the crease between the big toe and second toe on the left foot. Gently apply a light pressure and rotate the knuckle in a 'corkscrew' action so that it moves down the crease to the solar plexus reflex. Keep the knuckle in this position.

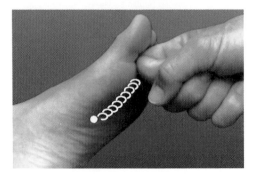

6 Gently press into the solar plexus reflex with the knuckle angled towards the inner aspect. Hold this compression to gain access to the small swelling that should 'pop out' at the side of the foot. This is the heart reflex which should be massaged very sensitively with the left middle finger in a clockwise motion; and then lovingly stroked.

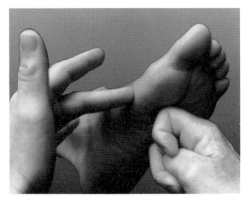

7 Remove the knuckle and make a fist with the same hand. Place this immediately below the ball of the left foot, with the knuckle in line with the diaphragm reflex. Use the right hand to rock the upper part of the left foot slowly and gently over the fist a few times.

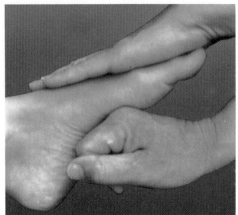

8 Feather stroke the whole reflex with light downward strokes, moving from lesser to greater.

9 Repeat all the steps on the right foot, reversing the roles of the hands. (If you find it difficult to 'corkscrew' with your left knuckle use the right one instead.)

Footnotes

- The breasts share the same reflex as the lungs. If you are concerned about any abnormal swelling or lumps in this area, professional advice should be sought to eliminate the possibility of breast cancer.
- Breasts represent maternal nourishment. Breast problems are associated with domineering attitudes, too much mothering and protection, or a complete denial of the nurturing process. A conflict of emotions arises between feeling restrained and a fear of developing.
- Concentrate on the diaphragmatic reflex to calm anxiety and return to the solar plexus reflex if the person feels panicky or asthmatic.
- Before moving from one task to another take time to close your eyes and be conscious of the expansion and contraction of your ribcage as you feel the breaths entering and leaving. If sounds or thoughts enter your mind, acknowledge them for what they are, recognise the feelings they evoke, and then return your attention to breathing. Do this repeatedly throughout the day for a few minutes at a time.
- Choose a specific time each day, such as in the bath or when lying in bed, consciously to take in deep breaths, hold them for a short while, then slowly squeeze all the air from the lungs. Hold this deflated feeling before taking in the next long, deep breath. Repeat 9 times.
- Take in the breaths of life lovingly and appreciatively. Enjoy the heady sensation of fullness and completeness.

The circulatory system

The circulatory system is an amazing logistical network, which furnishes nourishment and life to all parts of the body and transports energy for thought and action.

Position in the body
Blood circulates throughout the body with its centre, the heart, pulsating in the lower thoracic cavity, between the lungs.

Position on the feet
Circulatory reflexes are found extensively throughout the whole foot with the heart reflex at the base of the ball on the inner aspect of both feet.

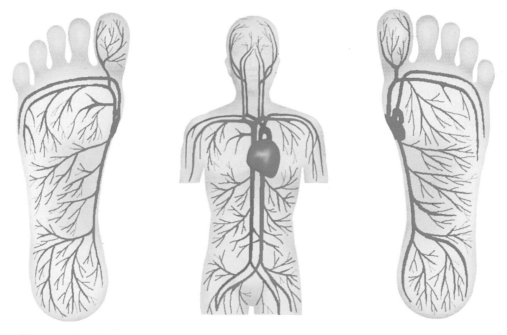

Characteristics

Blood circulates continuously in one direction around the body through an uninterrupted 60,000 mile network, over 1,000 times a day. It protects the body from harmful foreign substances, expels toxic wastes and prevents the body from bleeding to death in the event of injury. About 90,000 litres pass through the heart daily whilst distribution varies considerably in response to the ever-changing demands of the bodily systems. Blood vessels share the same lining as the heart, so that there are no joins or interruptions to hamper the smooth flow of blood.

Oxygenated blood courses through the arterial network from the left side of the heart to every part of the body to perform constructive and recuperative work. Broken-down material and wastes are then returned, through the venous network, to the right side of the heart before being transported to the lungs for the exchange of gases and other organs for the release of impurities. The rejuvenated blood returns to the heart to repeat the cycle. Veins have thinner, weaker walls than the arteries and contain valves to defy the laws of gravity.

Red blood cells outnumber white blood cells 500 to 1. They have a hectic but short lifespan of 120 days as they carry oxygen around the body. The larger white blood cells fight disease by digesting germs and only increase their numbers when there is an invasion of bacteria. The plasma acts as the transport medium of the body. Eight million cells die per second to be replaced by new ones from the bone marrow and lymphatic tissue.

The *heart*, a muscular organ with four chambers, is the centre of the circulatory system. Its two sides are completely separate but work in unison and harmony. The valves momentarily still the blood to allow the heart to assess the blood's ever-changing composition and contents. In this way the heart is constantly aware of inner and outer environmental changes so that it can control the balance and harmony between the two.

Effects of 'stress'

The respiratory and cardiac rates are closely related, and both respond immediately to activity and emotion. Physical activity increases the demand for vital forces, causing deeper breathing and faster heart beats. Emotions will either excite or depress the two systems depending on the interpretation and feelings experienced.

The width of the arteries, controlled by the nervous system, is drastically reduced during tension which imposes an incredible strain on the heart. The overworked heart endeavours to cope by pumping harder, which raises the blood pressure. If this continues indefinitely the heart weakens and may eventually enlarge. Deposits of fatty tissue on the walls of the blood vessels further reduce the lumen, compounding an already harmful situation. Cells are deprived of essential life forces and waste products dam up.

Excessive physical demands, environmental imbalances or exceptionally uninspiring situations damage the heart. Incorrect eating habits, extreme emotions and negative thoughts drain the heart of its courage and strength. An insufficient quantity of poorly digested food also affects the quality of blood and weakens the circulation.

Psychosomatic implications

The open-hearted person is like the left side of the heart, which generously gives of itself to others, whilst a close-hearted person is like the weary right side which continually stops to examine its contents. A soft-hearted person is filled with sentiment, whilst a hard-hearted person appears unmoved by emotion.

Diseases of the heart occur when it is drained of its enthusiasm and love, disturbing its synchronisation with life and nature. As the centre of love and emotion, any feelings of deprivation, as a result of long-standing emotional conflict, drains it of joy and vitality. Fear and anxiety grip it tightly, restricting its movements and causing a burning sensation. In the cold-hearted and hard-hearted, calcification occurs due to restricted mobility. Excessive consumption of alcohol and rich foods distort and abuse the heart, changing its shape and opening the way for inflammatory conditions. When love and joy are sacrificed and replaced by materialistic values and purpose, or life is believed to be traumatically filled with strains and distress, the heart becomes hardened and is prone to heart attacks.

Blood is the very essence and expression of love, which cherishes and supports each individual cell. When the vibrancy and quality of life are diminished, the impeded flow inhibits creativity and love. It may be physically barred by a blood clot or, as in anaemic blood, drained of its self worth and love due to a fear of life.

Varicose veins indicate a feeling of being over-burdened and trapped by a disagreeable life style, often accompanied by a hopeless discouragement.

High blood pressure occurs with long-term, persistent emotional problems.

Reflexology procedure

The circulatory system is extremely receptive to the gentle, loving, flowing massage of Reflexology. The blood vessel reflexes are throughout the foot and receive continual massage every step of the way. For the whole system to benefit, it is essential to massage the whole foot. The heart reflex was massaged with the respiratory tract (see page 62).

Footnotes
● It is advisable **not** to give a Reflexology massage to a person with a thrombosis since there is a risk that, as the body relaxes, the blood clot may dislodge itself and make its way to the brain or the heart.
● Enjoy life to the full with a loving attitude.
● Release all past unhappiness and bitterness.
● Select wholesome foods and eat correctly to allow your body to make the best blood and to service the specialised heart muscle.
● Exercise to keep the heart well toned and in shape.

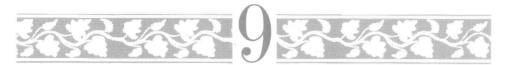

9

THE SPLEEN

The spleen produces blood cells, filters the blood, destroys worn out blood cells, serves as a reservoir blood supply and is believed to form antibodies.

Position in the body
On the left side of the abdomen, just below the diaphragm.

Position on the feet
The splenic reflex is present on the **left foot only**, immediately below the diaphragmatic reflex, towards the outer edge of the foot.

Characteristics

This fragile red organ is extremely soft and spongy covered by a fine elastic and muscular capsule. Although important, the body is able to function without it.

Reflexology procedure

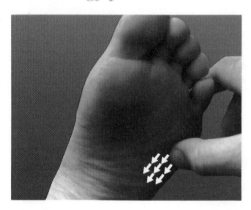

1 Caterpillar from the base of the diaphragmatic reflex to just above the waistline, along the outer edge of the foot. Continue to caterpillar in small vertical strips until you have covered the circular mound.

2 Milk the reflex, thumb over thumb.

3 Heal the area with downward strokes.

Footnote
● The splenic reflex swells and can be very sensitive during or just before an attack of malaria.

10

THE DIGESTIVE TRACT

Digestion is the remarkable process by which nutritional substances are converted and absorbed by the body to replenish and refuel cells, giving them vitality, quality and substance.

Position in the body
The digestive tract begins at the mouth, descends through the centre of the thoracic cavity to fill the bulk of the abdominal cavity, where it ends at the anus in the lower back.

Position on the feet
The digestive tract reflexes start halfway down the big toes and follow the inner aspect of the ball to occupy most of the fleshy instep. The rectum/anus reflexes curve round from the sole of the foot to the midway point between the ankle and heel on the inner aspect of both feet.

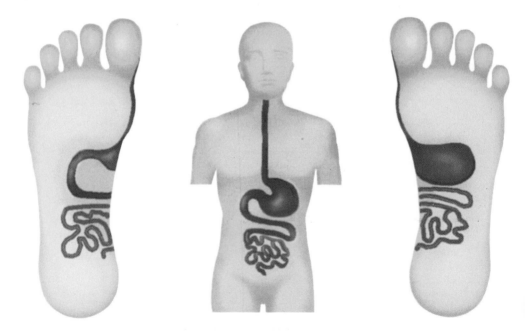

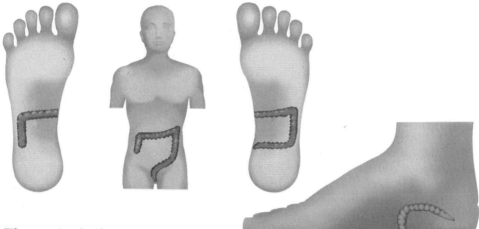

Characteristics

When supplies run low, hunger, one of the strongest desires, is detected by the brain and drives the body to seek fuel from food which, in its natural form, packages energy from the sun.

An amazing variety of food is consumed, but even in its most natural state it has to be processed into pure, simple elements, through the chemical activity of specific digestive enzymes, so that the most beneficial properties are extracted. This process, known as metabolism, is perfectly executed provided the correct amount of quality food is consumed under favourable circumstances.

Nutritional requirements   Each bodily cell has specific nutritional requirements depending on its position and function. Although the type of nourishment is of prime importance, it is even more crucial that the nutrients are metabolised correctly for digestion and absorption. The vitamin and mineral content of fruit and vegetables are sadly depleted by the time they are eaten, unless they are home grown for immediate consumption. Crops continually replenish their store of vitality whilst still growing but, once reaped, supply diminishes, just as a flower wilts after being picked. Thus it is necessary for the body to have vitamin and mineral supplements on a daily basis. Only natural foods provide a natural source of energy.

Effects of 'stress'

Although the digestive process cannot be controlled at will, it is heavily influenced by intense emotions such as anger, fear, excitement, tension and insecurity. Distress interferes with the release of hormones and enzymes, with a detrimental effect on the digestive process. Tension interrupts harmonious expansion and contraction, and hampers the food's digestion and causes cramping pain. The metabolic process is incomplete, malabsorption occurs, and the body is imperfectly nourished. Appetite is either depressed or increased.

Sadness, fear and depression dry the mouth, suppress gastric secretions, create an emptiness at the pit of the stomach and dull the system with heaviness. Aggression and resentment activate the gastric secretions despite lack of appetite and ulcerate the stomach's lining. Deprived of the tremendous amount of energy required for digestion, the system is without the strength or capacity to cope effectively.

Food is associated with comfort from early infancy when parents, unable to interpret the various crying signals, use feeding as a means of pacification often leading to obesity in later life. A baby may initially reject semi-solid foods since it may not be instinctively aware that it should swallow them. If this is interpreted as dislike, refined foods, which titillate and pamper the taste buds may be given instead, resulting in poor eating habits and 'fad' food addictions. These refined foods provide an immediate, short-lived boost of energy but have little or no nutritional value. The high intake of sugar, salts, colourants and preservatives is extremely detrimental to health.

Widespread social belief that set meals should be taken and the unnecessary intake of food burdens and over stretches the finely-tuned and precise system causing the overworked organs to store the excess as fat, further straining the body. Bolted food, improperly masticated (chewed) and insalivated, cannot be adequately digested.

Psychosomatic aspects

The digestive tract represents the taking in and absorption of life and vitality creating sustenance to provide physical and emotional strength and enthusiasm. Anorexia (compulsive starvation) cuts off these supplies due to deep fear, rejection, extreme guilt or self-hatred, whilst obesity provides a protective padding against the harsh realities of life. Fearful insecurity arises from self rejection, creating the need to seek fulfilment from food.

The power of Reflexology

Reflexology releases tension, re-establishes rhythmic motion, and allows food to be converted into an acceptable form for absorption and assimilation. Combined with sensible eating, weight can be controlled and vitality released.

Reflexology procedure

The soft abdominal cavity is reflected onto the fleshy instep of both feet.

There are two parts to the digestive tract:

1   The alimentary canal through which the food travels.

2   The accessory organs which play a major role in the digestive process but have no physical contact with the contents of the alimentary canal. These include the salivary glands, the pancreas, the liver and the gall bladder.

Digestive tract massage defies the principles of Reflexology!

Massage of all the glands, organs and canals, except the liver, follow the movement of the secretions and substances. If you can visualise the digestive tract on the foot it will simplify the procedure.

The accessory glands are attended to first. The salivary glands were massaged with the face and do not require further attention at this stage.

Footnotes

- Enjoy and appreciate eating the correct type and quantity of food that *your* body needs, when it is required.
- Energy from non-refined natural food is released at the optimum rate and provides substantial fuel and building material. Replenishment is required every 4 to 5 hours depending on the activity being pursued.
- The body is not equipped to manage the toxic 'foreign' substances found in colourants, preservatives and refined foods which may cause headaches and biliousness. It can be likened to giving diesel to a car that runs on petrol!
- Drink a glass of purified water when you wake up every morning, and then a further 7 or 8 glasses during the day depending on your needs. Avoid alcohol, caffeine and soft carbonated drinks.
- A house built with sub-standard material does not last. The body also needs to build solid foundations for health with the correct materials.
- The increased energy and quality of life gained from being aware of and meeting the nutritional demands of the body and mind far outweigh the possible scorn of others. They will learn to realise, appreciate and hopefully to emulate the energy and control of your life.

The liver

The liver is an extremely active organ with over 100 different chemical activities which generate much of the body's heat.

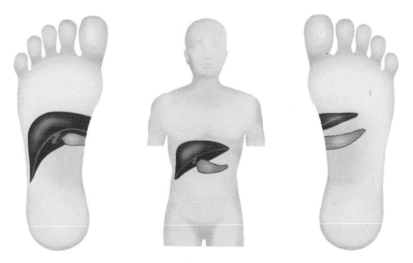

Position in the body
The liver is a roughly triangular shaped organ occupying most of the upper right hand corner of the abdominal cavity, immediately below the diaphragm.

Position on the feet
The liver reflex is mainly on the right foot where a triangular swollen mound occupies most of the outer half of the instep. The remainder of the liver on the left foot is massaged with the stomach reflex.

Characteristics

The liver is a solid, bright red organ with a spongy uniform texture. It is the largest and most versatile organ in the body. Over a litre of blood passes through its complex cells every minute although its greatest activity is at night when most of the body is resting. It has a multitude of responsibilities which it performs with exact precision and extreme proficiency.

Harmful substances such as alcohol, caffeine, nicotine and barbiturates are detoxified and substances in dangerous surplus in the blood, such as cholestrol, are modified. Large amounts of energy stored in the liver are continually depleted by the hungry brain and nervous systems which lack storage facilities of their own. It is a reservoir for blood; it synthesises proteins for blood clotting and destroys worn-out red blood cells after 120 days. Antibodies produced by the liver provide an essential defence against disease.

Bile, secreted by the liver and stored in the gall bladder, is released into the duodenum to neutralise acidic gastric juices and assist with the break down of fats. When expelled it influences the colour of the faeces.

Effects of 'stress'

The liver relies on a lush blood supply which, during stress, is significantly reduced and depletes the level of energy. Alcohol, nicotine, caffeine, barbiturates and all habitual means of coping with 'stress' place excessive strain on the nocturnal routine of the liver and increase the possibility of liver disorders.

Psychosomatic disorders

The liver represents the fiery seat of anger and the eruption of deep rooted emotions. Disorders indicate profound dissatisfaction and suppressed guilt believed to be justified through fault-finding in others.

Reflexology procedure

On the **right foot only**.

1 Find the triangular swelling that extends from the diaphragm reflex and tapers to a tip in the bottom left hand corner of the instep.

2 Caterpillar in vertical strips, from lesser to greater, with the left thumb until you have massaged the whole of the triangle.

3 Use the same thumb to milk downwards.

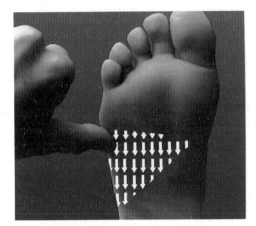
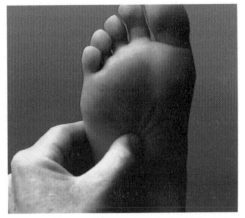

4 Locate the gall bladder reflex midway down the long side of the triangle. Place the thumb on this point and feel for a miniature 'sac'-like swelling.

5 Massage in a clockwise motion.

6 Press gently into the reflex, relax and release. (This reflex should still be massaged even if the gall bladder has been removed.)

7 Feather stroke the area with two fingers in a downward movement, from lesser to greater.

Footnote
● The liver reflex is extremely pronounced when detoxifying. When distressed it becomes swollen and taut. Any imbalances make it feel gritty, spongy or lumpy.

The pancreas

The pancreas is principally concerned with producing insulin, a substance that controls the metabolism of glucose in the body.

Position in the body
The pancreas nestles in the curve of the duodenum beneath the stomach.

Position on the feet
The pancreas reflex lies in the 'C' of the duodenum reflex (see page 78), immediately below the stomach reflex (see page 76) and above the 'waistline' of the foot.

Characteristics

The pancreas is a large tadpole-shaped gland which secretes glucagon and insulin into the blood stream. Glucagon and insulin enable the liver to release glucose, and insulin facilitates the use of glucose in all the cells of the body. The pancreas also pours about a litre of pancreatic juices into the duodenum each time the acid-laden food is expelled from the stomach, which chemically changes the duodenal contents.

Dysfunction of the pancreas Diabetes mellitus occurs if too little insulin is produced by the pancreas. The body's cells can't use the glucose in the blood and are therefore deprived of fuel. Stores of fat are used up and fatigue, weight loss, muscle wasting and tissue damage occur. If untreated, drowsiness, coma and eventually death can occur. Too much insulin reduces the blood-sugar levels alarmingly. The brain is deprived of glucose giddiness, sweating and extreme hunger are experienced. If untreated, unconsciousness, coma and eventually death can occur.

Psychosomatic aspects

The pancreas symbolises the pleasures and sweetness of life. It is thrown out of balance by feelings of rejection accompanied by the belief that life is void of delightful and enjoyable moments. This often occurs after a traumatic event, such as a divorce or the death of a loved one, and is exacerbated by anger and frustration.

Reflexology procedure

1 Rest the left thumb below the 'waistline' of the left foot, so that the upper edge of the thumb is in line with the 'waistline'.

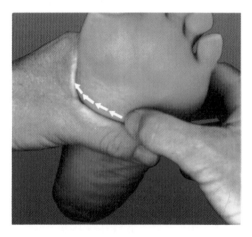

2 Use the right thumb to caterpillar from the edge of the splenic reflex along the horizontal strip immediately above the thumb. Repeat this movement over the same strip 3 to 4 times, moving from lesser to greater.

3 With the same thumb caterpillar vertically in minute strips from lesser to greater.

4 Milk the strip horizontally from lesser to greater as though squeezing the pancreatic contents towards the duodenum.

5 Feather stroke the reflex with two fingers using a light downward movement.

6 Move to the right foot.

7 Place the left thumb below the waistline on the right foot.

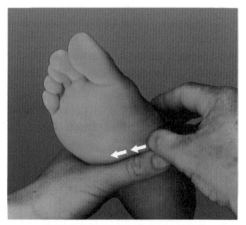

8 Use the right thumb to caterpillar horizontally across the strip immediately above the thumb from the instep to halfway across the right foot.

9 Caterpillar down in minute strips moving from greater to lesser.

10 Milk horizontally from greater to lesser, pushing the contents into the duodenum.

11 Heal (feather) the area gently downwards with both fingers.

Footnotes
- Diabetics should consult their doctor before having Reflexology massage. It is best to massage their feet *very gently* one hour before their insulin is due. The blood sugar should be tested before and after the massage since dramatic changes occur as the body attempts to stabilise and normalise the bodily processes.
- The pancreas is very sensitive to hunger and hypoglycaemia and feels tense, swollen and possibly gritty.

The oesophagus

The oesophagus channels food from mouth to stomach within seconds.

Position in the body
The oesophagus is the tube that connects the mouth to the stomach and runs through the centre of the thoracic cavity.

Position on the feet
The oesophagus is reflected onto the inner aspect of both feet from just below the centre of the big toes to the base of the ball.

Effects of 'stress'

Tension inhibits the rhythmic peristaltic waves causing a 'choked up' emotional feeling.

Reflexology procedure

1 Place the right thumb just below the centre of the inner aspect of the left big toe, with the thumb pointing downwards.

2 Caterpillar down to the base of the ball to where a protrusion can be felt, 2 to 3 times. Stop at this point and massage clockwise. Apply pressure, relax and release. This is the cardiac sphincter reflex.

3 Repeat the massage on the right foot with the left thumb.

Footnote
- The respiratory tubes share the same reflex so this area should also be concentrated on for any respiratory disorders, particularly asthma.
- Concentrate on the cardiac sphincter reflex for heartburn and hiatus hernia.

The stomach

The stomach transforms food by chemically and mechanically blending and homogenising it into a creamy substance known as chyme.

Position in the body

The stomach lies below the ribcage in the upper abdominal cavity with its bulk on the left side.

Position on the feet

The stomach reflex is predominantly on the left foot, immediately below the diaphragm reflex, occupying most of the upper part of the fleshy instep. The neck of the stomach is reflected onto the right foot, tucked beneath the diaphragm reflex.

Characteristics

The stomach is a thick-walled, elastic sac, controlled by involuntary muscle. It is relatively small but can expand to contain five litres. The stomach muscles contract approximately every three minutes during and after a meal and, even when empty, forcefully contract every 90 minutes or so with a rippling effect through the intestinal tract. Rings of muscle guard its openings – the cardiac sphincter at the entrance and the pyloric sphincter at the exit – to control the speed at which the stomach fills and empties according to the amount and type of food consumed.

Effects of 'stress'

Stress makes the stomach extremely sensitive to emotional fluctuations. Bursts of anger or excitement overactivate the muscles and agitate its lining which swells and turns scarlet. The increased secretion of hydrochloric acid is aggravated by chemicals, such as alcohol and aspirin, which destroy the protective coating and ulcerate the wall lining.

Conversely, its activity is dulled and its lining becomes pale and dry during periods of depression and extreme fear. An agitated cardiac sphincter allows some gastric contents to escape, which irritate the oesophageal lining and cause heart burn. A tense pyloric sphincter inhibits the release of stomach contents, producing a bloated, uncomfortable sensation. Abnormal eating habits impair normal functioning leading to fermentation and dyspepsia, gradually poisoning the whole system.

Psychosomatic aspects

The stomach helps to nourish and digest daily events. Resistance to the normal progression of life's circumstances, due to profound dread, extreme anxiety or fear of not being able to cope with new circumstances causes stomach upsets, particularly in young children beginning school or during examination time!

Reflexology procedure

1 Place the left thumb on the point immediately below the cardiac sphincter reflex and caterpillar horizontally, following the diaphragm reflex, to just beyond the solar plexus reflex.

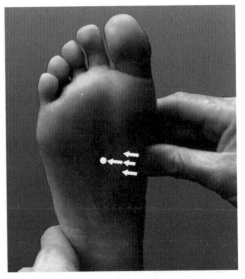

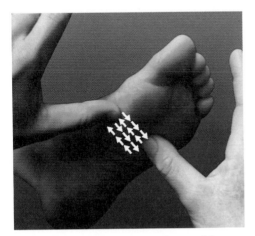

2 Place the right thumb on this point and caterpillar from lesser to greater over the same strip.

3 Repeat the 2 steps, from one side to another, as you churn the contents of the stomach reflex, ending with the right thumb on the inner aspect of the left foot.

4 Use both thumbs to milk the whole reflex, thumb over thumb, from lesser to greater.

5 Place the right thumb below the cardiac sphincter reflex on the right foot and horizontally caterpillar the neck of the stomach, from greater to lesser.

6 Finish with the thumb resting on the pyloric sphincter reflex, which can be easily felt as a slight swelling. Rotate clockwise. Gently press, relax and release.

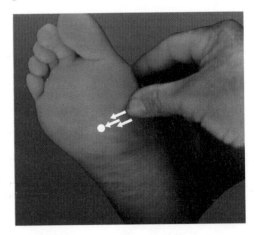

Footnote
● Concentrate on the stomach reflex during periods of extreme anxiety and uncertainty, and for any stomach disorders such as gastric ulcers.

The duodenum

Stomach contents are modified by the bile and pancreatic juices as the digestive process continues.

Position in the body
The duodenum is a short curved tube between the stomach and small intestine.

Position on the feet
The duodenum reflex follows a 'C' shape in the upper part of the right instep.

Characteristics

Small amounts of chyme spurt out of the stomach through a relaxed pyloric sphincter into the duodenum, which is the first part of the small intestine and the only section of the digestive tract that is more or less fixed in position.

Effects of 'stress'

Some acidic gastric juices escape through the tense pyloric sphincter ulcerating part of the duodenal lining. Tension prevents sufficient processing of the chyme leading to malabsorption.

Psychosomatic aspects

Duodenal ulcers indicate deep fear gnawing away at the insides, combined with a lack of self-confidence.

Reflexology procedure

1 With the right thumb still on the pyloric sphincter reflex on the right foot follow the 'C' of the reflected duodenum as it curves around the pancreatic reflex, making sure that you stay above the 'waistline'. You may need to change thumbs midway. Repeat this movement 2 to 3 times.

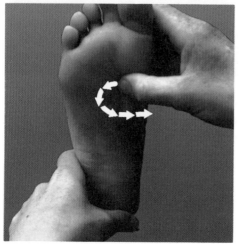
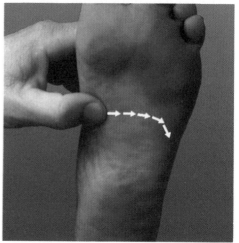

2 Continue to follow the duodenum reflex on the left foot. It is the strip immediately above the 'waistline' from the instep to the splenic reflex.

3 Keep the thumb in position ready to follow the small intestinal reflex.

The small intestine

Absorption of vital nutrients occurs in the small intestine.

Position in the body
The small intestine is ingeniously coiled into the confines of the lower abdominal cavity.

Position on the feet
The small intestine is reflected onto the lower half of both insteps.

Characteristics

The massive small intestine is remarkably free to expand and contract. Millions of minute finger-like projections, known as villi, increase its absorptive surface 600 times.

Effects of 'stress'

Tension irritates the nerves causing malabsorption and abdominal cramps. Centres of lymphatic activity are weakened by prolonged 'stress' opening the way to infection.

Psychosomatic aspects

The small intestine represents the ability to absorb the processes of life. Extreme fear or lack of self confidence block these natural processes, causing disease and discomfort.

Reflexology procedure

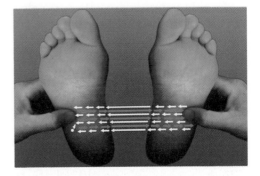

1 Continuing from the duodenal reflex make a loop, replacing the left thumb with the right thumb, so that the right thumb is ready to progress horizontally, from lesser to greater, in a line directly below the 'waistline'.

2 Take the right thumb over to the right foot to continue the line and caterpillar from greater to lesser as far as the colon reflex.

3 Allow the left thumb to take over from the right thumb to caterpillar along the horizontal strip immediately below the first, moving from lesser to greater.

4 Still with the left thumb, follow the strip through on the left foot until the colon reflex is reached.

5 Allow the right thumb to take over and continue to zig-zag backwards and forwards as you fill the lower half of the instep.

6 Finish the sequence with your right thumb poised on the ileo-caecal valve reflex situated only on the right foot.

Footnote
● Concentrate on this reflex for malabsorption and/or lowered immunity.

The large intestine or colon

Indigestible residues of digestion from the body are taken away for elimination by the colon to make way for fresh supplies of nutrients. The large number of resident bacteria produce important vitamins and amino acids.

Position in the body
The colon wraps around the small intestine in the lower abdominal cavity.

Position on the feet
The colon reflex outlines the small intestine reflex in the lower half of both insteps.

Characteristics

The large colon is shorter but three times as wide as the small intestine. It is puckered by bands of muscle to trap the massive build-up of gases, which are the end product of bacterial activity. The colon is most active between five and seven o'clock in the morning.

Effects of 'stress'

The solar plexus directly controls the colon making it extremely sensitive to emotion. Impending nerve-racking situations cause overactivity which, if prolonged, cause constipation.

Lowered immunity and the destruction of friendly bacteria by antibiotics increases the body's vulnerability to infection. Alcohol, certain chemicals and drugs also irritate the colon.

Psychosomatic aspects

The colon represents remnants of the past. An instilled dread of failure or deprivation of love and affection inflame and irritate the colon. Reluctance to release old beliefs, past emotions or material possessions can constipate the colon, whilst diarrhoea provides a form of escapism arising from a deep fear or feelings of rejection. A gripping fear, an inability to let go, or tension cramp the abdomen. Haemorrhoids indicate a dread of deadlines, congestion of old beliefs or a feeling of being encumbered and oppressed.

Reflexology procedure

1 Still with the right thumb on the ileo-caecal valve reflex on the right foot, feel for a tiny swelling very close to the ovary reflex.

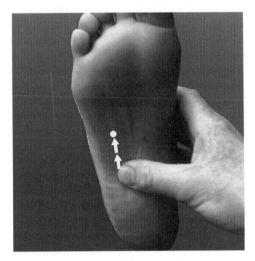

2 Rotate clockwise, press, relax and release.

3 Place the left thumb just below and fractionally to the left of the right thumb on the caecal/appendix reflex.

4 Caterpillar up the ascending colon reflex until you feel a

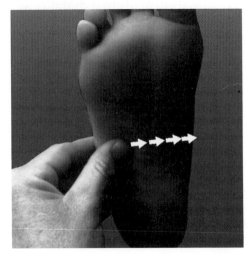

swelling either on or just below the 'waistline'. This is the hepatic flexure reflex. Massage this reflex in a clockwise direction. Turn the thumb 90 degrees to the right so that it is at right angles to the ascending colon reflex.

5 Caterpillar horizontally along the transverse colon reflex following the waistline to the edge of the inner sole.

6 Continue to caterpillar horizontally with the left thumb on the left foot, curving upwards slightly to the splenic flexure reflex where another swelling can be felt on the edge of the splenic reflex. Rotate in a clockwise motion, press and release.

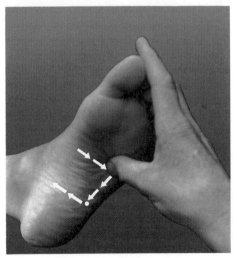

7 Now place the right thumb on this reflex so that it is facing downwards, then caterpillar down the descending colon to the base of the instep.

8 Turn the right thumb 90 degrees and caterpillar horizontally along the sigmoid colon which follows the base of the instep.

9 Keep the thumb in contact with the right foot as you caterpillar up the inside of the foot in a semi-circular curve to the anal reflex, in the slight hollow midway between the heel and ankle. Massage this reflex.

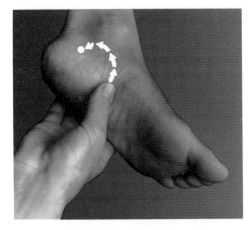

10 Place the left thumb on the inner aspect of the right foot and repeat the last movement.

Footnotes
● A tense ileo-caecal opening seems to prevent wastes from passing through to the colon from the small intestine. This has a detrimental damming effect and toxins are possibly absorbed into the blood stream, indicated by the extreme sensitivity of this reflex, particularly when there are allergies, asthma, skin irritations or nervous disorders.
● The hepatic and splenic reflexes are generally swollen, but may be tense if congested. Concentrate on the colon reflex for spastic colon, skin disorders, particularly acne, constipation, haemorrhoids, gastro-enteritis, diarrhoea, and ulcerative colitis.
● Include 3 fruits, raw vegetables and grains in the daily diet.
● Drink at least 6 glasses of purified water daily.
● Cough to release tension and to ease the expulsion of faeces from the rectum.
● Avoid the unnecessary administration of antibiotics. If they must be taken also consume some natural yoghurt.
● Release old constraining ideas and free yourself from constricting and often self-induced deadlines.
● Periodically have one day when only one fruit, either pawpaw, melon or grapes, is eaten to give the colon an opportunity to flush itself out. A clean colon encourages a more stable emotional life, whilst constipation leads to irritability and impatience.

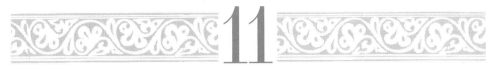

11
THE SKELETAL AND MUSCULAR SYSTEMS

The skeleton provides a rigid framework for the body allowing mobility.
It also protects vital organs.

Position in the body
The skeletal system is a mobile
frame clothed with muscles.

Position on the feet
There are skeletal and muscular
reflexes throughout the feet.

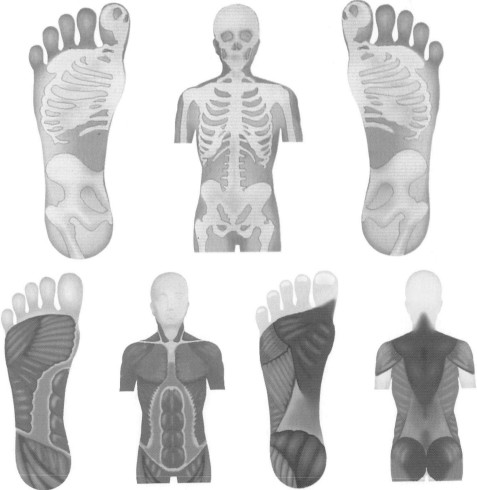

Characteristics

The shape of the skeleton was determined when humans began to stand upright over a million years ago. Over 200 finely balanced bones offer remarkable flexibility of movement despite the comparatively small size of the feet. With the skin it gives the body shape, strength and firmness to protect the delicate internal organs. Muscles, ligaments and joints facilitate a wide range of movement which allows thoughts to be put into action and the bodily expression of life's experiences.

Bones continually adapt to the physical demands of the body. They store important minerals to help maintain the correct chemical balance, whilst certain long bones manufacture red blood corpuscles for the circulatory system. The rate of development and eventual size of the bones is determined by the growth and sex hormones, as well as by the genetic make-up of families. Well co-ordinated activity ensures that muscles and organs adapt and adjust their size to keep pace with the growing skeleton.

Six hundred skeletal muscles determine the bodily form and are able to support 1000 times their own weight. These bundles of fibres are capable of contracting to almost half their original length. Their versatility and extreme sensitivity allow them to perform intricate and delicate tasks. They move with prodigious speed and power, generating an enormous amount of energy. The two other kinds of muscle in the body are the cardiac muscle, unique to the heart, and the involuntary muscles of internal organs and blood vessels. The automatic, unconscious movements of respiration, circulation, digestion, metabolism and excretion are never still. They require large amounts of fuel and oxygen, especially when active, after which the wastes need to be removed.

Effects of 'stress'

Distress alerts the body to impending dangers, real or imagined. Muscles contract and limit the range of movement, causing localised or general rigidity. Free expansion and contraction of the rhythmic cycles of respiration, circulation, digestion, and excretion are inhibited, depriving the cells of vital forces, with a subsequent build up of toxic wastes. The stiff muscular 'armour' causes 'dead' zones which prevent energy from coursing through the body.

Displaced bodily masses cause foot disorders and accentuate the spinal curve, upsetting the equilibrium. Spinal curvature compresses the posterior muscles of the lower back and distorts the physical alignment of the spinal column.

Bones under duress activate the body-building cells at the point of stress to strengthen and protect the area. This is particularly noticeable in the feet with the formation of bunions.

Skeletal development is adversely affected during prolonged periods of emotional 'stress' with reduced endocrinal activity hampering the production of growth and sex hormones.

Competitive sport can limit the body to learned gestures and encourage rigidity, with the use of aids like rackets and golf clubs repetitively straining the same muscles. Forced movements overtax an already stressed body to the detriment of the whole musculature. The pounding effect of high impact exercise on unnaturally hard surfaces ultimately impairs the joints.

Conversely muscles shrink and waste away if they are not used, depriving the body of mobility and heat.

The power of Reflexology

Stiffness in the foot represents stiffness in the body. Gentle manipulation and massage of the feet relaxes the body's musculature and releases it from the grip of deformity and strain. Physical performance is enhanced which, during sports, allows the body to ascertain its most natural and powerful movements. Relaxed muscles allow for freer bodily movement, versatility of all voluntary and automatic processes and the release emotional tension.

Psychosomatic implications

The skeletal structure represents the structural support of life, and the instinctive reaching out after things to turn them to one's own use. Emotional trauma and an exaggerated fear of injury cause the body to assume a stiff physical attitude to protect itself from anguish and pain. This resistance to power and authority causes brittle bones to break more easily. Deformities from the tight restraints of life limit the mobility of the mind and thoughts. Rage and obstinacy sprain the limbs and provide a physical excuse to avoid moving ahead in a particular direction. Joints allow flexibility and variety of movements, which influence and facilitate the course of life.

Reflexology procedure

Bone and muscle reflexes are continually being massaged throughout the whole Reflexology procedure. However, specific attention is given to the bones in the pelvic region, the arms and the legs (see pages 86, 91–92).

Footnote
● The Alexander technique, combined with Reflexology, helps to overcome deep rooted habitual misuse of the body which pulls it out of shape. It provides the practical tools to ease muscular tension and reduce damage to muscles and bones. The body can then work more energetically and competently in an unrestricted and natural way. (See Further Reading, page 127.)

The pelvic region

The pelvic tilt is important for the correct distribution of weight throughout the body. The hips help to maintain perfect balance and provide the tremendous force of forward mobility.

Position in the body
The pelvic bones support the lower abdominal cavity with the pelvic muscles forming a floor at the base.

Position on the feet
The pelvic region is reflected onto the heels of both feet.

Characteristics

The pelvis is a sturdy framework which snugly articulates the leg bones and provides attachment for the major leg muscles. It keeps the body vertical and protects part of the small intestine, the bladder, the reproductive organs and other internal structures. The sciatic nerve passes through the hip to the thigh.

The pelvic bones are held firmly together by ligaments which soften during pregnancy so that the pelvis is more flexible during childbirth.

Effects of 'stress'

Tension causes rigidity and limits mobility. The sciatic nerves can sometimes become trapped, resulting in excruciating pain from the base of the spine to the ankle. During childbirth tension prevents the free expansion of the pelvic cavity, narrows the birth canal and increases the amount of energy required for the expulsion of the baby which leads to unnecessary pain and trauma.

Psychosomatic implications

Hip problems indicate a reluctance to step forward because the future looks bleak or provide a physical means of avoiding implementation of important decisions. This can be temporarily brought about by grief over personal loss, or by depression as a result of traumatic events.

Sciatica can either arise from hypocritical behaviour or a deep concern about financial and future developments.

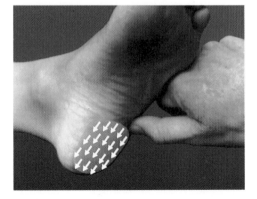

Reflexology procedure

1 Use the right thumb to caterpillar vertically down the left heel, moving from lesser to greater.

2 Milk with firm downward movements.

3 Gently heal the reflex with feathery downward strokes, using two fingers.

4 Repeat the massage on the right foot with the left thumb.

Footnote
● The skin on the heel can be very tough in which case a little more

pressure may be necessary.
● Cracked ankles should receive attention and a pedicure would be advisable. The daily application of natural balms and creams will help to soften the area and prevent the heels from cracking. Concentrate on this reflex for sciatica and any pelvic or hip disorders.

The lymphatic 'J'

The lymphatic vessel reflexes are massaged at this stage to flush out toxic substances from the sides of the body.

Position in the body
These lymphatics are on the sides of the body.

Position on the feet
These lymphatic reflexes follow the perimeter of the foot from the base of the little toe, along the side of the feet and around the heel.

Reflexology procedure

1 Place the right thumb at the base of the little toe on the left foot with the thumb facing downwards.

2 Caterpillar down the perimeter of the foot making sure that you are on the bottom, and not at the side of the foot.

3 Stop when you have finished the 'J' shape around the heel. Repeat two to three times.

4 Milk the area in a downward strip.

5 Feather stroke, using tiny downward strokes with two fingers.

6 Repeat the above steps on the right foot using the left thumb.

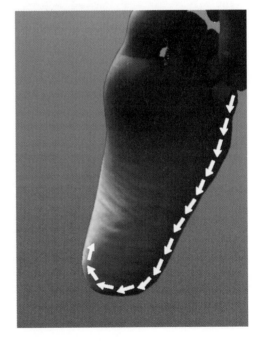

Upper lymphatics

The toxic wastes from the head and arms accumulate in the shoulder region and these reflexes now need to be massaged.

Position in the body
These lymphatic vessels extend from the head to the base of the neck and over the shoulders.

Position on the feet
These reflexes are in between the toes.

Reflexology procedure

1 Caterpillar with the right little finger going through the gap between the fourth and fifth little toes on the left foot, from the bottom of the foot to the top.

2 Milk through the gap in the same direction.

3 Repeat steps 1 and 2 through all the spaces between the toes on the left foot until you reach the big toe.

4 Repeat on the right foot with the left little finger.

Footnote
● Concentrate on these reflexes for any head or neck congestion and disorders. Also for tense shoulders.

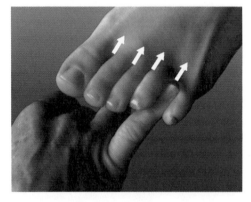

The back and the neck

The back provides flexibility, support and protection, particularly to the organs situated in the torso. The neck gives flexibility and agility to the head allowing the sensory organs to scan the environment.

Position in the body
Across the back of the neck and body.

Position on the feet
On top of both feet, the neck is reflected onto the neck of the toes and the back from the base of the toes to the ankle.

Psychosomatic implications

Back problems indicate a weakness in the support system (see page 28).

Reflexology procedure

1 Gently squeeze the left toenails, from the left little toe to the left big toe.

2 Rest the sole of the left foot against the open left hand.

3 Caterpillar with the right thumb in vertical strips from the tip of the little toe to the ankle crease 2 to 3 times.

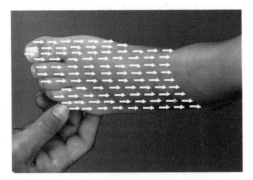

4 Continue to caterpillar each vertical strip from the tip of every toe to the ankle crease, 2 to 3 times each, massaging from lesser to greater until the spinal reflex is reached.

5 Place 4 fingers either side of the foot and, with the left fingers, caterpillar, with all 4 fingers, horizontally across the top of the left toes and foot from greater to lesser. As you reach the outer edge repeat with the right fingers

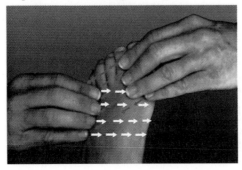

massaging from lesser to greater. Continue this movement up to the ankle crease.

6 Use the heel of the right hand to milk the whole area, starting at the little toe.

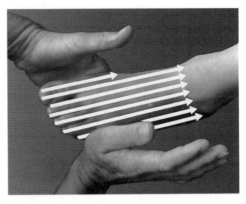

7 Gently feather stroke the whole area with all your fingers towards the ankle.

8 Repeat all the above steps on the right foot with the left thumb and hand.

Footnotes
• The top of the foot can be extremely sensitive and needs to be massaged very gently. A spongy feeling, particularly over the upper region, may indicate internal crying or a feeling or being burdened. Concentrate on the shoulder reflex for those who feel weighed down by responsibilities.
• The back reflex also provides secondary access to the lung and breast reflexes.
• Lie down with the knees bent, breathe deeply, relax and gently press your back flat against the floor. Also try to straighten the neck. Do this for a few minutes every day to remind your back of its correct position.

● Stand and sit tall and erect at all times. Pull your torso out of the hips, and your neck away from the shoulders. You should feel lighter and more alert. The correct posture and structural alignment relieves strain on internal organs and releases tension. It activates the mind and energises the body.
● 'Responsibility' means 'the ability to respond', and need not be burdensome.

The limbs

The limb systems provide an active means of survival and present the mind, body and spirit with the opportunity to experience new situations which in turn feed the mind with progressive ideas. The limbs are in constant communication with the rest of the body and provide food to refuel and energise the body's mobility.

Position in the body
The limbs are mobile projections from the upper and lower part of the human torso.

Position on the feet
The legs are reflected, in fetal position, on to the outer side of both feet. The arms reflexes also appear on the external edge of the feet.

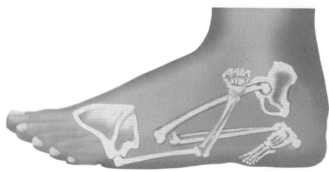

Effects of 'stress'

Muscular deformity of the body causes abnormal rotation of the feet. Flat feet are the result of internal rotation of the knees. Corns and callouses indicate protest against the abnormal distribution of bodily weight. Shoes can constrain, more than protect, feet.

Psychosomatic implications

The limbs represent the mobility of thoughts and life. Feet carry an image of the self and symbolise our connection with life processes whilst hands represent our capacity to handle and deal with life's experiences. Thigh problems indicate a reluctance to release traumatic past events, whereas disorders of the lower leg indicate a resistance to progress forwards.

Reflexology procedure

1 Place the right thumb on the bony prominence (shoulder reflex) at the base of the left little toe. Massage gently in a clockwise motion.

2 Caterpillar up the edge of the left foot to the bony protrusion (elbow reflex) midway along the outer side of the foot and massage with a clockwise motion.

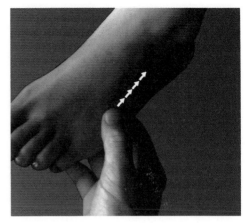

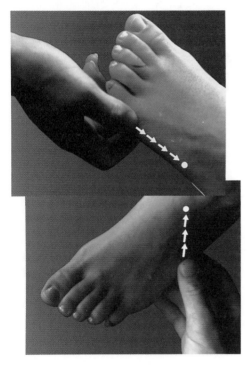

3 Change the direction of the thumb so that it is pointing up towards the upper end of the bony hollow at the base of the outer left ankle bone.

4 Caterpillar until you find a bony swelling (hand reflex) and massage gently.

5 Lift the right thumb and place it on the outer edge of the left foot, midway between the shoulder and

elbow reflexes, but fractionally higher than the upper arm reflex. This is the knee reflex which feels like a bony ridge.

6 Direct the thumb so that it is pointing towards the lower end of the bony hollow at the base of the outer ankle bone.

7 Caterpillar up to the base of the left ankle to the ball-like swelling which represents the hip joint. Massage this reflex gently but well.

8 Raise the left leg supporting the ankle in the left hand and caterpillar, with the right thumb, in strips towards the body until the triangular portion of the outer heel is completely massaged.

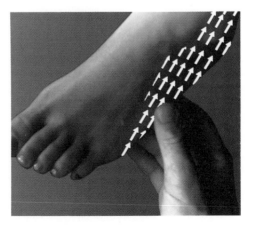

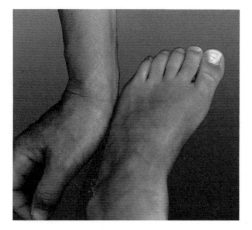

9 Milk and heal with the heel of the right hand.

10 Repeat on the right foot with the left hand.

Footnote
● An extra bone in the body is reflected as an extra bone in the foot. Crushed bones or injuries can also be detected. To respect and preserve the perfect morphology of the feet choose your footwear carefully. The soles of shoes should be completely flat, to allow the foot to adapt itself to the ground, and to maintain the body's alignment.

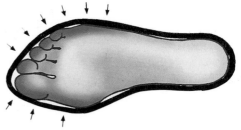

The thoracic cavity

Position in the body
The thoracic cavity, or mediastinum, is situated between the chest and upper back.

Position on the feet
The mediastinal reflex is the fleshy area between the upper part of the bony spinal reflex and the 'waistline'. The heart, lungs, main blood vessels, respiratory and digestive tubes and nerve centres are all contained within the theoracic cavity.

Reflexology procedure

1 Caterpillar 2 to 3 times, with the right thumb, from the base of the left big toe, along the fleshy instep to the 'waistline'.

2 Milk towards the heel.

3 Heal the area stroking towards the body.

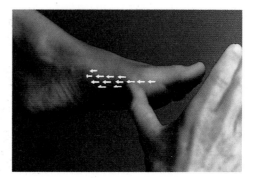

4 Repeat on the right foot with the left thumb. The heart, lungs, main blood vessels, respiratory and digestive tubes and nerve centres are all contained within the thoracic cavity.

Footnote

● Concentrate on this area for any heart or chest problems, or for deep anxiety.

12

REPRODUCTIVE ORGANS

The ability of living things to reproduce their kind is a miracle of nature. The human race survives to reproduce, and reproduces to survive. From an early age the instinctive awareness and attraction between sexes increases the possibility of reproducing new individuals based on existing patterns.

Position in the body

The *male* reproductive organs are suspended below the abdomen.

Position on the feet

The *male* reproductive organs are reflected onto the inner aspect of both ankles.

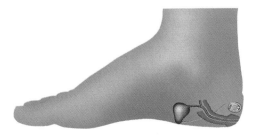

The *female* reproductive organs nestle within the deep confines of the pelvic region in the lower abdominal cavity.

The *female* reproductive organs are reflected onto the soles as well as the inner aspect of the instep. They can also be approached from the outer heel and over the crease of the ankle.

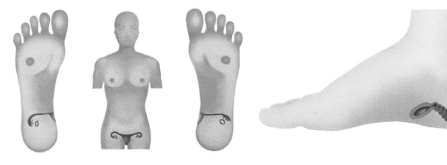

Characteristics

The male testes produce the hormone testerone which determines
development of the male characteristics, involving a range of physical
changes in puberty: a tremendous growth spurt, an increase in the size of
the reproductive organs, the presence of facial and bodily hair and the
deeper voice, all of which make the male more attractive to the female
and thus increase his chances of sexual activity. The descent of the two
testes, with their hundreds of metres of tubing, into the hanging scrotum
provides ideal cooler conditions for the production of sperm. From the
onset of puberty the male is capable of ejaculating 200 million sperm
every 24 hours until old age!

The female body has been purpose-built for the reproductive process.
Whilst in the womb, the female foetus has approximately 7 million ova,
many of which degenerate leaving only a million or so at birth, of which
only 300,000 are present at the menarche (onset of periods). A mere 400
or so will mature during the reproductive years. Fertilisation of two ova
occurs in 80 percent of pregnancies, and these develop until the third or
fourth month, after which the weaker one is absorbed. The womb
attempts to reject any foetus that is abnormal, or if bodily conditions are
inadequate, accounting for the large number of miscarriages, many of
which are never known by the woman.

The remarkable uterine muscle is the only muscle that, once
contracted, never regains its original length. This causes the womb to
shrink during childbirth for the natural expulsion of the baby.

Effects of 'stress'

The sexual physiological changes and new social pressures often create
confusion and strain during puberty. The hormonal secretion is
extremely susceptible to fluctuating mood changes, which in turn creates
turmoil as the reproductive cycles develop.

Inhibiting social and religious beliefs as well as pornographic material
create confusion about sexuality and give it a lewd, mysterious slant, with
bizarre, inhibiting and occasionally abusive ideas developing. These
distort natural appreciation and admiration for the magnificent human
form and obscure the development of human expression through loving
relationships. Fear of expressing deep, innermost feelings, combined
with the inability to discuss sexuality openly, even between partners, has
dire physical and emotional consequences. Tension, with its vice-like
grip, creates unconscious barriers and inhibits the reproductive flow,
interpreted as rigidity, infertility, impotence, menstrual and
reproductive disorders and diseases.

If the muscles of virginity, which extend from the pubis down the
inside of the thighs, are consistently tense they will cause foot
deformities.

Menstruation, pregnancy and childbirth are as natural to the female
body as digestion and respiration, but preconceived ideas and the high

level of muscular rigidity, distress the body and create an endless list of common complaints, such as dysmenorrhoea (painful periods), amenhorroea (abnormal absence of periods) and nausea, preventing the full enjoyment of sexual processes.

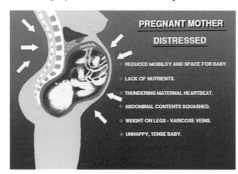

PREGNANT MOTHER
DISTRESSED

- REDUCED MOBILITY AND SPACE FOR BABY.
- LACK OF NUTRIENTS.
- THUNDERING MATERNAL HEARTBEAT.
- ABDOMINAL CONTENTS SQUASHED.
- WEIGHT ON LEGS – VARICOSE VEINS.
- UNHAPPY, TENSE BABY.

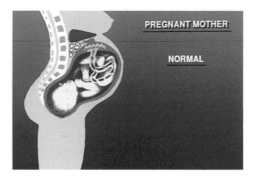

PREGNANT MOTHER

NORMAL

The power of Reflexology

If the feet are massaged from birth, the body is able to develop naturally. The nervous and endocrine systems are sufficiently balanced to allow full sexual development with a natural expression of love.

The menstrual flow can be flushed through calmly and effectively, pregnancy and childbirth become the enjoyable and awe-inspiring experiences that they should be, and babies are calmer, healthier and happier for their less traumatic experience.

Ideally both partners should receive regular Reflexology massage and consciously feed their bodies wholesome, natural sources of essential nutrients. Toxic substances should be avoided for at least a year prior to conception, to reduce the incidence of miscarriages, deformity and infertility (provided there is no mechanical problem). This regime should continue throughout pregnancy and labour to enable the body to relax totally and to ensure the natural development of the fetus in a harmonious environment. After birth Reflexology encourages the body to return to its natural state and gives the parents the strength to cope lovingly with the persistent demands of the baby.

Psychosomatic implications

The reproductive system speaks the language of love and creativity. If sexuality is believed to be sinful and 'dirty' or if reproductive processes are considered to be an inconvenience and a burden instead of a natural and necessary phenomenon, physical barriers and imbalances occur.

The sexual glands and parts of the reproductive organs were stimulated with the massage of the endocrine system. To massage the remaining sexual organs, particularly for the male:

Reflexology procedure

1 Place your right thumb on the 'waistline' on the inner aspect of the left foot and caterpillar towards the heel.

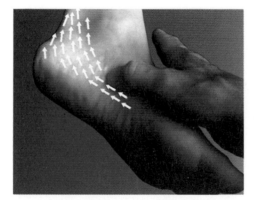

2 Using the 'waistline' as the starting point each time, continue to caterpillar up the foot until you have completed massaging the triangular area below the left inside ankle.

3 Milk and heal the heel area.

4 Gently lift the left foot with the left hand and lightly grip the left heel between 2 right fingers.

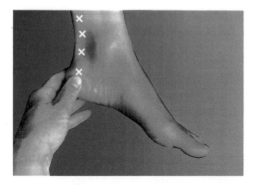

Caress the heel, first by gently pinching it, moving up towards the body and then lightly squeezing it between the 2 fingers.

5 Repeat the whole sequence on the right heel.

Footnotes
- Pregnancy can be detected by a foetal shaped swelling in the uterine reflex on the side of the foot.
- A Reflexology massage can be administered during menstruation. The menstrual flow is no more toxic than uric or faecal wastes. Massage should, however, not be given by someone who is irritable due to pre-menstrual tension.
- Men should avoid wearing tight trousers or having hot baths, both of which adversely affect the production of sperm.
- Women should avoid vaginal deodorants.

Posterior lymphatics

The lymphatics are massaged at this stage to accumulate all toxic wastes from the neck, shoulders and back reflexes and to flush them into the actual lymphatic vessels situated in the feet.

Position in the body
Widely distributed throughout the back and buttock regions, with concentrations in the groin.

Position on the feet
These reflexes are found throughout the top of the feet with concentrations around the ankles.

Reflexology procedure

1 Caterpillar from the outer base of the little toe, following the edge of the ligament, to the ankle crease. Milk immediately.

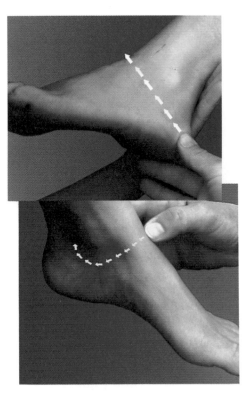

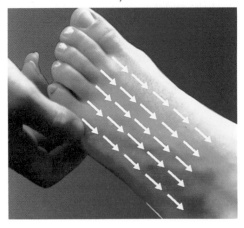

2 Repeat this movement between every ligament, from the gap between each toe to the ankle crease, until you complete 5 strips.

3 Place the right thumb on the outer tip of the left heel pointing upwards.

4 Caterpillar along the crease, over the top of the ankle, under the inner ankle bone and then up along the edge of the ankle so that your thumb ends up at the upper, posterior tip of the ankle bone. Repeat 2 to 3 times and then milk and heal.

5 Now caterpillar with the left thumb from the inner tip of the left heel to below the inner ankle and up the edge of the ankle bone to the anterior tip of the ankle bone. Repeat 2 to 3 times before milking and healing.

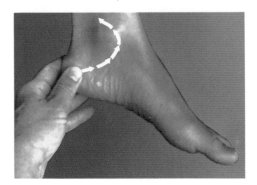

6 Place the right thumb at the base of the outer left heel and caterpillar up either side of the ankle bone. Repeat a couple of times and then milk and heal.

7 Repeat the above sequence on the right foot, reversing the role of the hands.

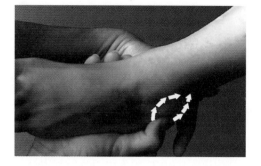

Footnotes
- Massage thoroughly if congested, and for back, hip or pelvic disorders.
- The strip over the ankles is a secondary reflex area for the fallopian tubes in females.

13

THE URINARY TRACT

Kidneys cleanse the blood of poisons and soluble impurities and help
regulate water and mineral balance.

Position in the body
The kidneys are firmly attached to
the posterior wall of the abdomen,
slightly above the waistline. The
ureters descend through the
abdominal cavity to the bladder,
which nestles at the base of the
pelvis.

Position on the feet
The kidneys are reflected onto the
soles of both feet, just above the
'waistline', with the right kidney
being slightly more central and,
due to the liver, fractionally lower
than the left. The ureter reflexes
extend from the kidney reflex,
through the instep, to the bladder
reflex, which is the small swelling
on the inner aspect of the foot at
the base of the instep.

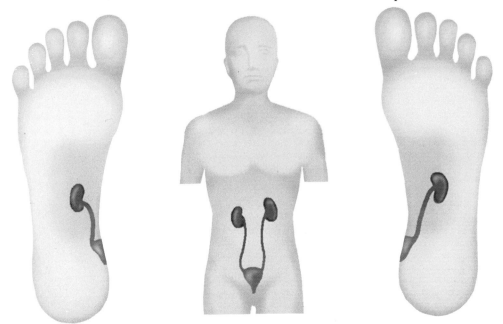

Characteristics

The correct volume of fluid in the body involves delicate interplay
between the brain, kidneys, lungs and skin. The task of eliminating

surplus water requires discriminating separation of the many useful chemicals in the blood, such as nutrients, hormones and minerals, from the waste products. The two kidneys cope admirably and only require one third of their tissue to work well.

Thirst, one of the strongest desires, arises from the high concentration of salts in the blood. The body can survive only two to three days without water. A five percent loss of water triggers the need to drink; ten percent leads to illness, and 20 percent to death despite over 30 litres remaining in the body. Most people, however, drink far more than is necessary.

Every day the total blood volume passes 300 times through the kidneys which monitor, filter and process approximately 1000 litres of blood with incredible speed and efficiency, from which only one litre of urine is produced.

Several hormones, which detect changes in the water content of tissues and trigger the kidneys into action, prevent flooding or dehydration.

Effects of 'stress'

Tension inhibits the activity of the urinary tract and reduces the amount of blood flowing through it, leading to water retention and bloatedness. Certain drug molecules clog the miniscule tubules, which then collapse. The effects are not immediately felt because two thirds of the tissue are not essential but, ultimately, kidney failure can occur. Pressure and negativity during childhood can lead to bedwetting. Bacteria and viruses make their way from the outside world, through the stressed bladder and ureters, into the vulnerable kidney, particularly in females due to the proximity of the vagina and because they have a significantly shorter urethra than males. Physical trauma to a full bladder during the descent of the baby at childbirth can stretch and weaken the urethra causing incontinence and possible prolapse in later life unless post natal exercises are undertaken.

Psychosomatic implications

Kidney problems arise from severe disillusionment, criticism or lack of success, which cause the person to revert to childish behaviour. Urinary infections commonly occur in those who are 'fed up' with their partner, or who continually hold others responsible for their misfortunes.

Reflexology procedure

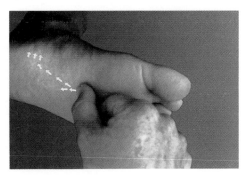

1 Place the right thumb on the left adrenal reflex and gently rotate in a clockwise manner.

2 Keeping the thumb on the reflex, alter the direction of your thumb so that it is facing directly downwards.

3 Caterpillar the kidney reflex a few times before caterpillaring along the ureter reflex into the bladder reflex. Caterpillar the whole bladder reflex, working towards the body before caterpillaring along the urethra to midway between the inner ankle and heel. Massage this point.

4 Milk and then heal the whole area before moving onto the right foot.

5 The right adrenal reflex is fractionally lower and closer to the instep than the left one.

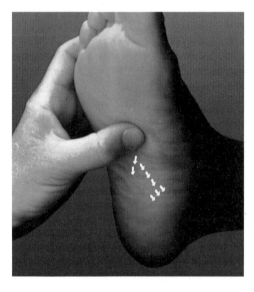

Footnotes

● Concentrate on the urinary reflex for any urinary or eye disorders, as well as for water retention. Many people wish to urinate as soon as this reflex has been massaged. For this reason, it is left until the end.

● All females should do daily pelvic floor exercises, particularly after having babies, to prevent prolapse of the uterus and bladder and to avoid incontinence later in life. Cross your legs whilst lying or standing and squeeze the pelvic muscles, by pulling them up into the body, and hold; squeeze them further and hold; then squeeze them even more and hold. Remember to breathe at the same time!

● Never take diuretics for weight loss or fluid retention, unless specifically prescribed by a doctor when they **must** be taken with a potassium supplement.

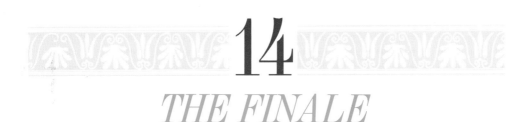

14

THE FINALE

To finish the massage

1 Gently but firmly **pull** all the toes progressively starting with the little toes simultaneously and then the next pair until you reach the 2 big toes. If necessary stand, to get your weight behind the toes, and keep pulling, especially for migraines, neck stiffness and back problems. It is similar to putting the head in traction.

2 Individually **rotate** each toe, anti-clockwise and then clockwise, starting with the left little toe and finishing with the right big toe.

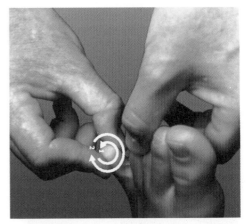

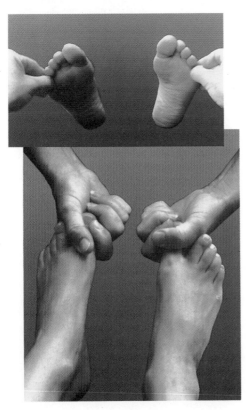

3 Place both hands in alignment on top of both feet and then **stretch** them downwards.

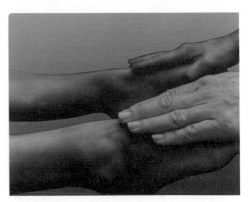

Place the hands under the feet to **push** them upwards.

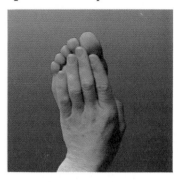

4 Placing the hands either side of the foot, manipulate and **rock** the feet from side to side.

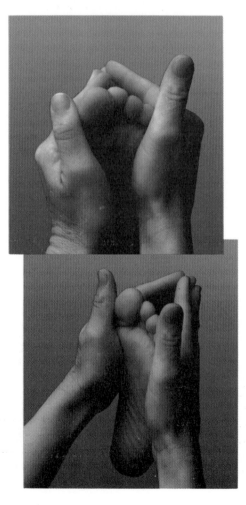

5 Supporting the left foot in the left hand, **rotate** the whole foot with the right hand, first anti-clockwise and then clockwise, making sure that you gently stretch it to its limit.

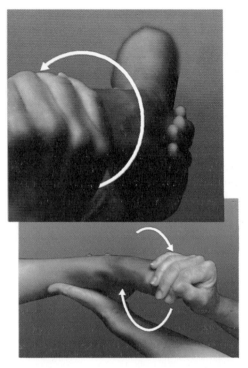

6 With fingers on top of the foot and thumbs underneath, **open** the left foot by pulling gently downwards with the fingers, starting near the toes and finishing at the ankle. Repeat on the right foot.

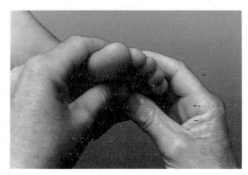

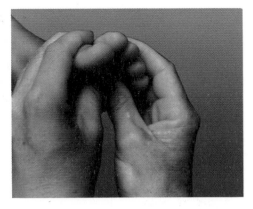

8 Gently feather the whole left foot from the tip of the toes to the heel, starting on the sole. Repeat on the right foot.

9 Finish with the solar plexus massage for at least a minute (see page 30).

7 Grip the left big toe between the 2 hands and twist one hand up and one hand down – similar to a 'Chinese bracelet' to manipulate the spinal reflex. Gradually move the hands along together to the 'waistline'. Do not go beyond this point – the spine has no flexibility in this region.

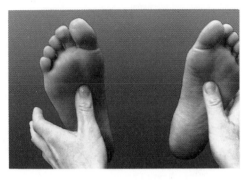

10 Cover the feet with the sheet or blanket.

Footnote
● The recipient should continue to relax for a short while before getting up slowly, and if sleeping, they should be left. Give them a large glass of purified water and encourage them to drink further glasses for the next 24 hours to flush out toxic substances.

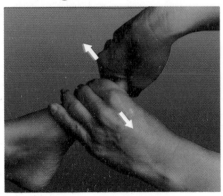

Reflexes on both Feet

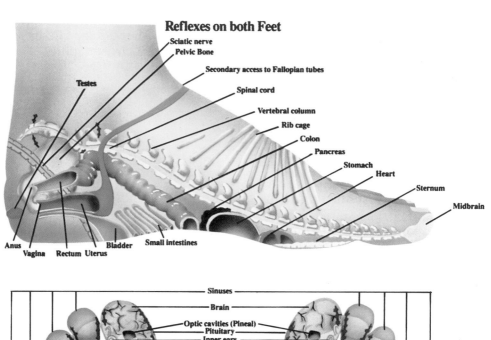

Sciatic nerve
Pelvic Bone
Secondary access to Fallopian tubes
Spinal cord
Vertebral column
Rib cage
Colon
Pancreas
Stomach
Heart
Sternum
Midbrain
Testes
Anus
Vagina   Rectum   Uterus
Bladder
Small intestines

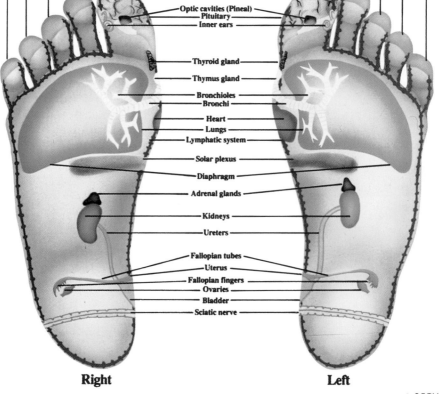

Sinuses
Brain
Optic cavities (Pineal)
Pituitary
Inner ears
Thyroid gland
Thymus gland
Bronchioles
Bronchi
Heart
Lungs
Lymphatic system
Solar plexus
Diaphragm
Adrenal glands
Kidneys
Ureters
Fallopian tubes
Uterus
Fallopian fingers
Ovaries
Bladder
Sciatic nerve

Right   **Left**

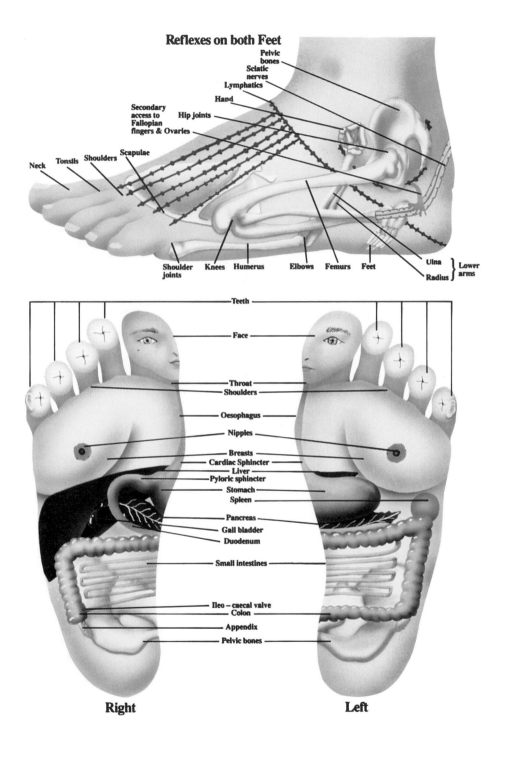

Reflexes on both Feet

Pelvic bones
Sciatic nerves
Lymphatics
Hand
Secondary access to Fallopian fingers & Ovaries
Hip joints
Neck
Tonsils
Shoulders
Scapulae

Shoulder joints
Knees
Humerus
Elbows
Femurs
Feet
Ulna
Radius } Lower arms

Teeth
Face
Throat
Shoulders
Oesophagus
Nipples
Breasts
Cardiac Sphincter
Liver
Pyloric sphincter
Stomach
Spleen
Pancreas
Gall bladder
Duodenum
Small intestines
Ileo – caecal valve
Colon
Appendix
Pelvic bones

Right   **Left**

15

STEP BY STEP SUMMARY

Always massage the left foot first and then the right.

The warm up

Stroking

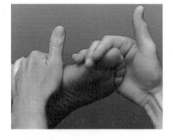 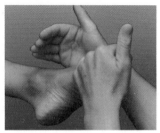

Circle the ankles

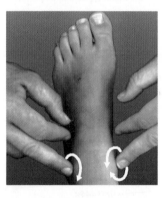

Ankle shake

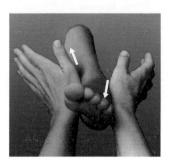 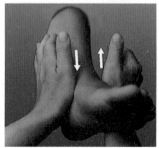

Foot rub

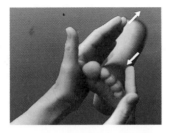

Achilles stretch

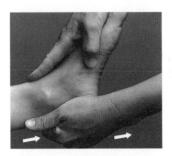 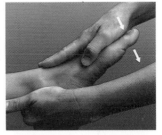

Knuckle rub

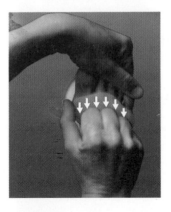 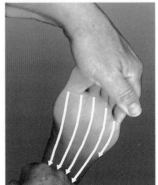

Spinal rub

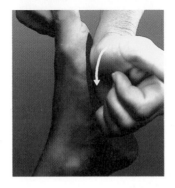

The central nervous system

Caterpillar down, milk and heal the left big toe.

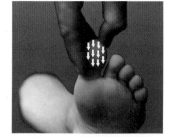

Repeat on the right **brain** and **face** reflex.

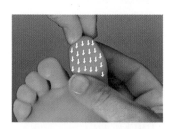

Caterpillar in 3 strips, milk and heal towards the body.

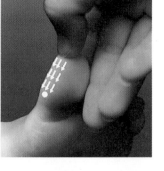

Repeat on the right **mid-brain** reflex.

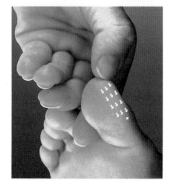

Caterpillar in 3 strips, milk and heal towards the body. Repeat on the right **neck (cervical)** reflex.

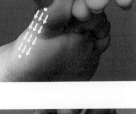

Caterpillar 3 strips. One under the bone, one immediately on the bone, and the last over the bone. Milk and heal all 3 strips. Repeat on right **spinal** reflex.

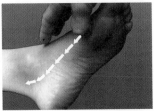

Stroke the whole reflex with the third finger from the tip of the left toe to the ankle. Repeat on the right foot.

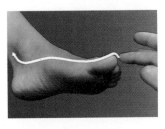

Place both thumbs on the two **solar plexus** reflexes simultaneously and gently press. Hold for up to 5 minutes.

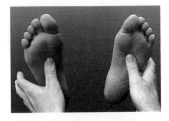

The endocrine system

Place thumb on left **pituitary** reflex. Rotate, press in gently and slowly release. Repeat on right reflex. Balance.

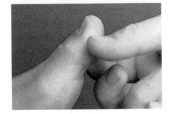

Rotate, gently press and slowly release the left **pineal** reflex. Repeat on the right reflex. Balance.

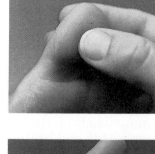

Rotate, press, and release the left **thyroid** reflex. Repeat on the right reflex. Balance.

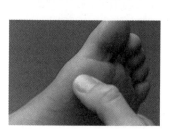

Rotate, press and release the left **thymus** reflex. Repeat on the right reflex. Balance.

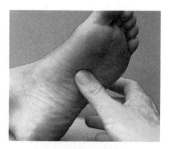

Rotate, press and release the left **adrenal** reflex.

Repeat on the right **adrenal** reflex, which is slightly lower and more towards the instep. Balance.

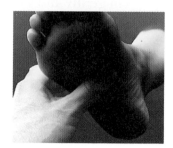

Rotate, press, and release the left **ovary** reflex. Repeat on the right reflex. Balance.

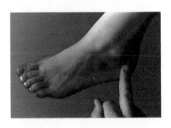

Rotate, press and release on **high stress (ovary)** reflex. First on the left and then the right. Balance.

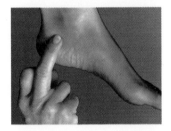

Rotate, press and release the left **prostate (vaginal)** reflex, and then the right. Balance.

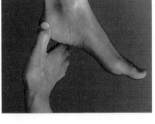

Press, rotate and release the left **testes (pubic bone)** reflex, then the right. Balance.

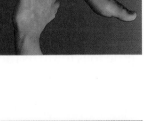

Sinus, teeth, eyes, ears, nose and throat

Rotate, press and release the left **inner ear** reflex. Repeat on the right. Balance.

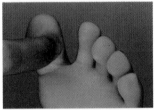

Caterpillar down each little toe, moving from the little toe towards the big toe. Milk and heal. Repeat on right foot. These are the **sinus**, **teeth**, **eye** and **ear** reflexes.

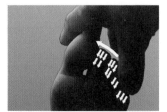

Caterpillar down the neck of each toe, concentrating on the neck of the big toe. Milk and heal. Repeat on the right **throat** reflexes.

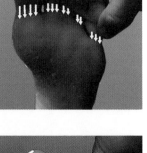

Squeeze down the sides of each toe to drain the **lymphatics**.

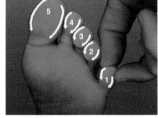

Upper lymphatics

Caterpillar across the base of the little toes towards the gap between the big and second toes.

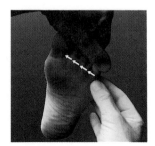

The respiratory and cardiac systems

Caterpillar down the ball of the left foot and then milk.

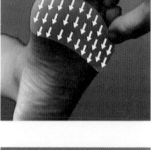

'Corkscrew' down the crease to the solar plexus reflex.

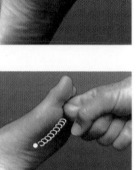

Press gently into the solar plexus reflex to 'pop out' the heart. Massage the **heart** reflex.

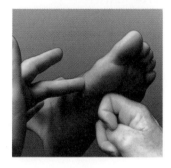

Place the right fist under the left **diaphragmatic** reflex and bend the upper foot over the fist several times. Massage the **diaphragm** reflex.

Repeat all 4 steps on the right **chest (breast)** reflex.

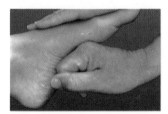

The spleen

Caterpillar down, milk and heal
the **splenic** reflex. On *left* foot only.

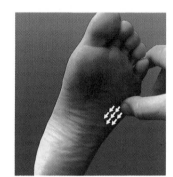

The digestive tract

Caterpillar to fill in the triangular **liver** reflex
on the *right* foot only and then milk and heal.

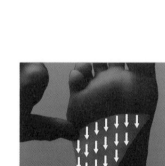

Gently massage, press and release the **gall
bladder** reflex.

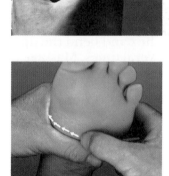

Caterpillar across the left **pancreas** reflex, milk
and heal.

Caterpillar from greater to lesser along the right **pancreas** reflex.

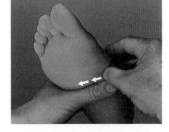

Caterpillar down the left **oesophagus** reflex to the **cardiac sphincter** reflex. Massage this reflex. Repeat on the right foot.

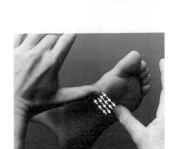

Massage the left **stomach** reflex with both thumbs, moving from side to side, and finish with the left thumb pointing towards the right foot.

Caterpillar the right **stomach** reflex from greater to lesser.

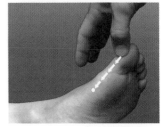

Massage the **pyloric sphincter** reflex.

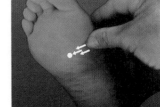

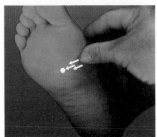

Caterpillar around the 'C' of the **duodenum** reflex on the right foot.

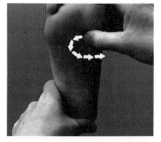

Continue to follow this reflex on the left foot. Caterpillar horizontally, from one foot to the other, across the **small intestinal** reflex.

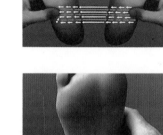

Massage the **ileo-caecal** reflex. Caterpillar up the **ascending colon** to the **hepatic reflex**.

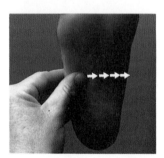

Massage the **hepatic flexure**, turn the thumb and caterpillar along the **transverse colon** reflex moving from the right to the left foot to the **splenic flexure**.

Massage the **splenic flexure** reflex, turn the thumb down and caterpillar down the **descending colon** reflex. Turn the thumb again to caterpillar along the **sigmoid colon** reflex.

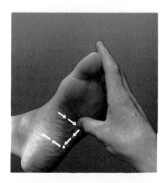

Caterpillar the **rectum** and massage the **anal reflex**.

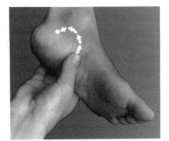

Milk the entire alimentary canal and then both insteps. Finish by healing the whole area.

The skeletal, muscular and lymphatic systems

Caterpillar down, milk and heal the left and then the right **pelvic** and **sciatic** reflexes.

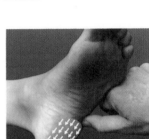

Caterpillar, milk and heal the **lymphatic 'J'** reflexes on the left and then the right foot.

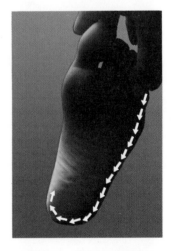

Caterpillar and milk through the toes, first on the left and then on the right foot.

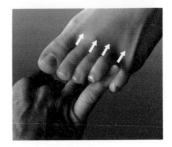

Squeeze toe nails, then caterpillar from the tips of the toes to the ankle crease. Milk with the heel of the hand and heal. Repeat on the right foot.

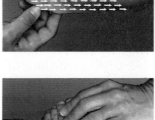

Four finger massage with both hands across the tops of both feet.

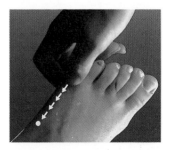

Massage the **shoulder socket** reflex and then caterpillar to the **elbow** reflex. Repeat on the right foot.

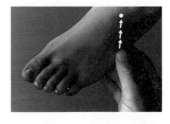

Massage the **elbow** reflex and then caterpillar up to the **hand** reflex. Repeat on the right foot.

Massage the **knee** reflex and then caterpillar up to the **hip socket** reflex. Repeat on the right foot.

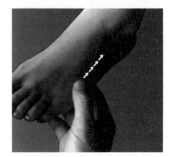

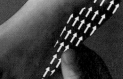

Caterpillar, milk and heal the outer left ankle. Repeat on the right **leg** and **buttock** reflexes.

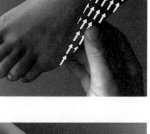

Caterpillar, milk and heal the **mediastinum** reflex, first on the left and then the right.

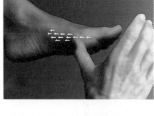

Caterpillar, milk and heal the left inner ankle, and then the right **reproductive** and **pelvic organ** reflexes.

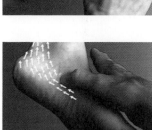

Raise the left leg and gently 'pinch' and then lightly squeeze the left heel. Raise the right leg and repeat.

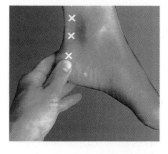

Massage and milk the 5 left **lymphatic** strips and then the right.

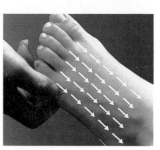

Caterpillar and milk
the left **lymphatic**
reflex over the ankle
crease and around the
inner ankle.

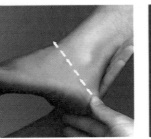
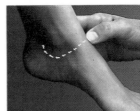

Caterpillar from top of left inner heel up to
left inner ankle. Repeat on right foot.

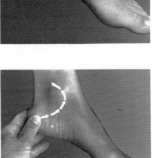

Caterpillar and milk the outer left ankle and
repeat on the right **lymphatic** reflex.

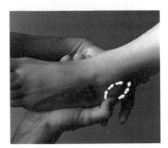

The urinary system

Massage, milk and
heal the **kidney**,
ureter, **bladder** and
urethra reflexes first
on the left foot and
then on the right.

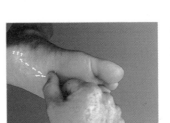
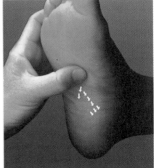

The finale

Pull toes

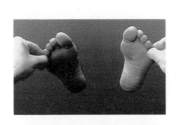 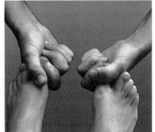

Rotate toes

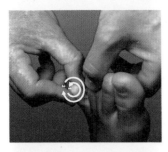

**Stretch down and
then up**

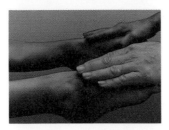

Rock the feet

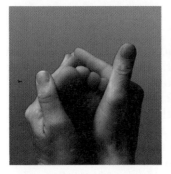 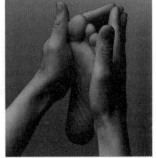

Rotate foot

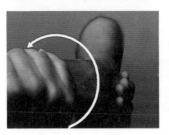 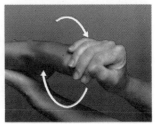

Open foot

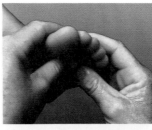 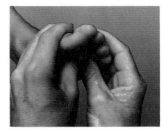

Spinal twist

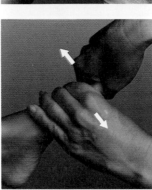

Solar plexus for at
least a minute

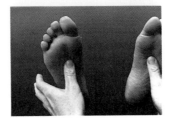

Self administration

Whilst self administration is feasible, there are obvious limitations, not the least of which is difficulty in achieving the relaxed posture so essential to experiencing full benefit! However, specific discomfort such as a headache or stomach ache can be temporarily relieved.

Simple but effective therapy can be achieved by walking barefoot whenever possible. Greatest benefit is induced by a walk without shoes in the relaxing environment of a sandy shore or on grass along the banks of a river. Such idyllic conditions are seldom readily available but in less favourable conditions, all is not lost. A few minutes of rolling a golf ball or fluted bottle between foot and floor is better than no therapy at all!

Whatever the circumstances, it is important to create a relaxed environment devoid of stress and one most conducive to relaxation. You may prefer absolute quiet whilst someone else finds that soft soothing music helps. It is easier to feel restful when your surroundings are neither too hot or too cold. Adopt a comfortable posture and, before massaging your feet, take time to let go, physically and mentally. Relax, with this handbook nearby, and revel in the release you will feel.

16

THE WHOLISTIC APPROACH TO HEALTH

> 66 *The challenge is great. The rewards are greater.* 99

In this book emphasis is placed on the coined word 'wholistic' rather than on the conventional 'holistic' in order to avoid the implications which the latter spelling tends to attract. Although Reflexology is a powerful means to develop and maintain a healthy body it is but part of the wholistic approach. For the best results, 'the whole' – mind, body and soul which by nature are one – must be addressed whilst other forms of therapy have their part to play. According to individual requirements, these may include Aromatherapy, Shiatsu, Herbadology, Acupuncture, Homoeopathy and so on.

Reflexology procedures aim directly to correct physical imbalances within the body and, indirectly, emotional imbalances. It will be obvious to the reader that the latter calls for greater effort on the part of the recipient than of the giver. Attitude and an open mind play a significant role.

In the course of time as therapy proceeds, its tranquil effect takes care of the emotional aspects so that the mind becomes increasingly receptive. It is then easier to replace negative by positive thought and extremes by moderation.

The benefits gained from Reflexology, practised in accordance with this handbook, are legion but reach their zenith within an appropriate environment. The benefits of therapy are soon dissipated by a life-style lacking balance. It may be necessary to modify long standing habits, be they to do with diet, drink, smoking, dress and so on, to achieve a state of equilibrium conducive to a healthy and rewarding life. The responsibility rests with the recipient. The challenge is great. The rewards are greater. Step out and begin to appreciate life.

Life is precious – guard it;
Life is a challenge – meet it;
Life is tense – ease it;
Life is a promise – keep it;
Life is a pleasure – enjoy it;
Life is rough – smooth it;
Life is a duty – do it;
Life is life – live it.

Anon

FURTHER READING

Alexander Technique; Headway Lifeguides: Glynn MacDonald; Hodder & Stoughton, London

Attitudinal Healing, Dr Andrew Cooks; from his own notes, Johannesburg

Anatomy and Physiology for Nurses, Sheila Jackson; Bailliere Tindall, International

Blessed by Illness, L F C Mees, MD; Anthroposophic Press, New York

Body, The, Life Science Library; Time-Life International (Nederland) NV

Body Book, The, Reader's Digest; Reader's Digest Association, International

Brain: A User's Manual, The, The Diagram Group; Berkley

Hand and Foot Reflexology, Kevin and Barbara Kunz; Thorsons Publishing Group, London

Healing through Colour, Theo Gimble, DCE; The Burlington Press, Cambridge

Health Building, Dr Randolf Stone, DO, DC; CRCS Publications, United States of America

Illustrated Physiology, McNaught and Callander; Longman Group Limited, New York

Iridology, Farida Sharon, MD, (MA), MH, ND, FBRI; Thorsons Publishing Group, London

Language of the Feet, Chris Stormer; Hodder & Stoughton, London

Living Body, The, Karl Sabbagh with Christian Barnard; Macdonald and Company Limited, London

Living With Your Body, Walter Buhler; Pharos Books, London

Perfect Health, Deepak Chopra, MD; Bantom Books, International

Reflex Zone Massage, Franz Wagner, PhD; Thorsons Publishing Group, London

Reflexology: The Definitive Guide, Chris Stormer; Hodder & Stoughton, London

Seeing Beyond 20/20, Dr Robert-Michael Caplan; Beyond Words Publishing, Hillsboro

Star Healing, David Lawson; Hodder & Stoughton, London

Way Your Body Works, The, Dr Bernard Stonehouse; Mitchell Beazley International Limited, London

Whillis's Anatomy and Physiology, Roger Warwick, BSc, PhD, MD; J and A Churchill Limited, London

Yoga: Headway Lifeguides, Mary Stewart; Hodder & Stoughton, London

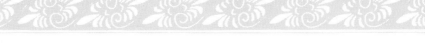

USEFUL ADDRESSES

Bayley School of Reflexology
Monks Orchard
Whitbourne
Hereford and Worcester
WR6 5RB
Tel: 01886 21207

British School for Reflex Zone Therapy of the Feet
97 Oakington Avenue
Wembley Park
London
HA9 8HY
Tel: 0181-908 2201

British School of Reflexology
PO Box 34
Department NH
Harlow
Essex
Tel: 01279 29060

Metamorphic Association
67 Ritherden Road
London
SW17 8QE
Tel: 0181 672 5951

Midland School of Reflex Therapy
5 Church Street
Warwick
CB34 4AS
Tel: 01926 491071

Raworth Centre
20/26 South Street
Dorking
Surrey
Tel: 01306 742150

Hoths School for Holistic Therapy
39 Prestbury Road
Pittville
Cheltenham
Gloucestershire
GL52 2PT

Mary Martin School of Reflexology
37 Standale Grove
Ruislip
Middlesex
HA4 7UA
Tel: 01895 635621

Larger College of Reflexology
41 Parkfield New Ross
County Wexford
Ireland
Tel: 0151 22209

House of Healing
87 The Lookout
Chepstow
Gwent
NP6 5BL
Tel: 012912 6064

Crane School of Reflexology
135 Collins Meadow
Harlow
Essex
CM19 4EJ
Tel: 01279 21682

Lillian Stoltenberg School of Holistic Reflexology
96 Pennsylvania Road
Exeter
Devon
EX4 6DQ
Tel: 01392 219798